This book is dedicated to my dear friend Pat Clutter, who set the example for me to be willing to take the risks to follow my dreams and "think outside the box". Pat has not only set the example, but has been kind enough to share leads and opportunities for me to be able to follow my own dreams. Pat has bravely followed me on crazy adventures not only in nursing but all around the world. Her companionship, mentorship, and friendship have helped shape me into the emergency nurse I am today.

Thanks Pat!

Author's Note

I suspect that many people will use this pocket book as a study guide to prepare to take the Certification in Emergency Nursing Exam (CEN)® . I am certain this can be a valuable tool for that goal. I highly recommend that the pocket books be used to <u>augment</u> preparation for the exam. These books were not written or designed as the sole tool for studying. They should instead be used to re-enforce and solidify knowledge gained from more complete sources. The "pearls of wisdom" within this book may sometimes contain concepts or words that the reader may be unfamiliar with. Seize that opportunity to seek out more information about the concept or word so that the "pearl" makes sense. By doing that, the reader can maximize their learning potential. Good luck in your endeavors.

Jeff Solheim

Table of contents

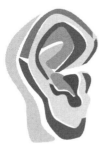

Maxillofacial
Emergencies

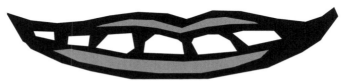

- Ⓟ The first cranial nerve is the olfactory nerve and is responsible for the sense of smell.
- Ⓟ The second cranial nerve is the optic nerve and is responsible for vision.
- Ⓟ Temporal arteritis is an inflammation of the blood vessels of the temporal artery.
- Ⓟ Ludwig's angina is an infection of the submandibular, submental, and sublingual spaces. The infection spreads from dental infections involving the second or third molar.
- Ⓟ A loose tooth is also known as a subluxed tooth.
- Ⓟ Patients with a temporomandibular joint dislocation will have significant discomfort and difficulty speaking or swallowing. The mouth may be partially open and the patient may drool.
- Ⓟ The fifth cranial nerve is the trigeminal nerve and it has motor functions (chewing and clenching the jaw) and sensory functions (sensation of the face.)

- ⓟ A disorder of the fifth cranial nerve is known as trigeminal neuralgia. The common name for this disorder is Tic Douloureux.
- ⓟ Trigeminal neuralgia results in excruciatingly painful electrical shock-like sensations along the jaw line, the cheek, and sometimes into the forehead area.
- ⓟ Patients with an anterior epistaxis will have blood loss from the nares, whereas patients with a posterior epistaxis are more likely swallow and vomit blood.
- ⓟ Otitis externa is an infection in the external auditory canal and auricle of the ear.
- ⓟ Labrynthitis is an infection of the inner ear. It may be caused by a bacterial or viral infection, ototoxic medications or have an auto-immune cause.
- ⓟ The seventh cranial nerve is the facial nerve and it has motor functions (allows movement of the face) as well as sensory functions (allows taste).

- ℗ A disorder of cranial nerve seven is known as Bell's Palsy.
- ℗ Bell's palsy causes a unilateral loss of facial movement and diminished taste.
- ℗ Sinusitis is a common diagnosis that is caused by various bacteria infecting the mucosal lining of the paranasal sinuses, most frequently the maxillary sinus.
- ℗ Always consider the possibility of vertebral and intracranial injuries when caring for patients with facial trauma.
- ℗ Common mechanisms of injury associated with mandibular fractures includes assaults, falling forward on the chin, and motor vehicle collisions.
- ℗ Cervical spinal injuries, intracranial injuries, and basilar skull fractures are all associated with facial fractures.
- ℗ Clear drainage from the nose following head trauma should be tested with a glucose strip. Cerebrospinal fluid is high in glucose, but nasal discharge is not.

- Ⓟ The best position to assess for a fractured zygomatic arch is at the head of the bed, looking down at the arches with the health care provider's eyes level to the patient's forehead.

- Ⓟ Patients with Ludwig's angina carry the potential of airway obstruction due to edema and accumulation of secretions in the mouth.

- Ⓟ Patient's with minimally subluxed teeth may be discharged home on a soft diet for two weeks, allowing the dental ligaments to re-tighten.

- Ⓟ Sore throats caused by a virus are often accompanied by cough and nasal discharge.

- Ⓟ Sore throats caused by a bacteria have a more rapid onset of symptoms than viral sore throats, and are usually accompanied by a higher fever then is found with a viral sore throat.

- Ⓟ A frequent cause of epiglottitis is *Hemophilus B*. Immunizations now exist for this bacterium, reducing the incidence of epiglottitis, especially in the pediatric population.

- ℗ Both posterior and anterior epistaxis may lead to varying degrees of hypovolemia, but a posterior epistaxis often carries a higher risk for significant blood loss.
- ℗ Meniere's disease is a fluctuation of fluid in the inner ear that often occurs between the fourth and sixth decade of life.
- ℗ Foreign bodies in the external ear canal may be removed using forceps, hooks, loops, or irrigation with a syringe and saline.
- ℗ Rare, but serious complications of sinusitis include orbital cellulitis, orbital abscesses, epidural abscesses, subdural abscesses, meningitis, brain abscesses, cavernous sinus thrombosis, and osteomyelitis of the frontal or maxillary bone.
- ℗ Lacerations of the eyelids should be repaired as soon as possible before swelling commences and the borders cannot be adequately matched.
- ℗ Patients with trauma to the neck carry a high risk of airway obstruction.

Ⓟ A LeFort I fracture is a fracture of the maxilla that causes detachment of the maxilla above the teeth but below the nose, creating a free floating palate.

Ⓟ A LeFort II fracture is a fracture of the maxilla over the bridge of the nose resulting in a free floating mid-face.

Ⓟ A LeFort III fracture is a complete detachment of the facial bones from the skull.

Ⓟ Symptoms associated with zygomatic fractures include paresthesia of the cheek, nose, and upper lip, with subcutaneous emphysema of the face, as well as periorbital ecchymosis, and unilateral epistaxis.

Ⓟ Factors which may contribute to Bell's palsy include emotional stress, viruses affecting the nerve such as the Herpes Simplex virus, or cold drafts to the face.

Ⓟ Temporal arteritis causes severe stabbing pain in one or both temples. The patient may also experience increased pain when chewing.

Ⓟ Pericoronitis is an inflammation of the gingival tissue surrounding the crown of a tooth.

Ⓟ An Ellis class one tooth fracture is a fracture through the enamel portion of the tooth. The tooth will appear chalky white and may appear jagged.

Ⓟ Croup is most common in the fall and early winter.

Ⓟ Causes of an anterior epistaxis include nose picking, dry air, infections, trauma, local irritants, foreign bodies, anticoagulant drug therapy, hypertension, bleeding disorders, recreational drug use, and tumors.

Ⓟ The same factors which can cause an anterior epistaxis can cause a posterior epistaxis. The only exception is nose picking because the finger cannot extend to the posterior nasopharynx.

Ⓟ Causes of otitis externa include bacteria, viruses, fungi, perforation of the skin in the ear canal, foreign bodies or skin conditions such as eczema in the external ear canal.

- Ⓟ Both labrynthitis and Meniere's disease cause tinnitus as well as nausea and vomiting.
- Ⓟ Ellis class one tooth fractures are not considered emergent and are treated as needed for cosmetic reasons on an outpatient basis.
- Ⓟ Bread and vegetable matter in the external ear canal should not be flushed with saline as this will soften them and make removal more difficult. These substances are removed dry with a suction tip or blunt instrument.
- Ⓟ Symptoms of sinusitis include nasal congestion, mucopurulent nasal discharge, malaise, fever, facial swelling, and pressure over the involved sinus.
- Ⓟ Airway should always be a consideration and priority when caring for a patient with maxillofacial trauma.
- Ⓟ Clinical manifestations of tracheal and/or laryngeal trauma includes dyspnea, hemoptysis, subcutaneous emphysema, dysphonia, and loss of thyroid prominence.

Ⓟ Ocular entrapment is recognized by movement of one eye while the other eye remains fixed. This is a sign of an orbital fracture.

Ⓟ Have the patient with an anterior epistaxis blow their nose, than lean forward in the seated position, tilt their head downward and pinch the nostrils as close to the nasal bones as possible.

Ⓟ The patient with an anterior epistaxis should pinch their nostrils a minimum of ten minutes continuously without releasing pressure.

Ⓟ Otitis externa starts with itching in the ear canal followed by pain in the canal that may radiate to the head, jaw and neck. The pain is worse with external manipulation of the ear.

Ⓟ Otitis media is frequently associated with upper respiratory tract infections, but may also occur secondary to barotrauma.

Ⓟ Labrynthitis causes sensitivity to noise on the affected side,

Ⓟ Meniere's disease causes mild to severe hearing loss on the affected side.

- Ⓟ Continuous bubbling in a patent chest drainage system is one possible indication of upper airway or bronchial trauma with internal air leakage.
- Ⓟ Malocclusion, where a patient's teeth don't fit together properly, is a sign of a mandibular fracture.
- Ⓟ If cerebrospinal fluid (CSF) leakage is suspected in bloody drainage from the ears or nose, allow a drop of blood to fall on a gauze square. If CSF is present, a yellow ring will form around the blood on the gauze. This is sometimes called the "halo test".
- Ⓟ Cranial nerves three (oculomotor), four (trochlear) and six (abducens) are responsible for movement of the eye.
- Ⓟ Patients with Bell's palsy may experience pain in the occipital area of the head as well as behind the ear on the affected side.
- Ⓟ Patients with temporal arteritis will complain of pain when the side of the face and forehead is palpated.
- Ⓟ Viral sore throats are self-limiting and must run their course.

Ⓟ An Ellis class two tooth fracture is a fracture that extends through the enamel into the underlying dentin. The tooth will take on a yellowish appearance.

Ⓟ An Ellis class three tooth fracture extends through the enamel and dentin, exposing the underlying pulp and nerve. These fractures are extremely painful.

Ⓟ Significantly subluxed teeth should be referred immediately to a dentist to salvage the tooth and to reduce the risk of infection.

Ⓟ Bacterial sore throats are frequently caused by beta-hemolytic streptococci and are commonly referred to as "strep throat."

Ⓟ Croup causes a sore throat. The condition causes an exudate to be discharged from the throat that is irritating to the vocal cords causing a harsh, barky cough.

Ⓟ Anterior epistaxis not controlled by direct pressure may require the application of local vasoconstrictors such as 2% or 5% cocaine hydrochloride or Neo-Synephrine.

- Ⓟ Monitor for systemic hypertension when caring for a patient who has had a local vasoconstrictor applied to control an anterior epistaxis.
- Ⓟ Patients with otitis externa may complain of hearing loss and a feeling of fullness in the canal due to swelling of the external auditory meatus.
- Ⓟ Infants and children who are pre-verbal may "tug" at their ear as an indication of otitis media.
- Ⓟ Labrynthitis causes lateral dizziness, Meniere's disease causes rotational vertigo.
- Ⓟ LeFort fractures should be cared for with the head of the bed elevated when possible.
- Ⓟ The paralysis of Bell's palsy usually resolves within several weeks or months.
- Ⓟ Temporal arteritis may cause the blood vessels in the temple of the affected side to become red, swollen and tortuous.

Ⓟ Pericononitis is associated with erupting teeth, impacted teeth, or accumulation of food or bacteria in the gums.

Ⓟ Common mechanisms that may precede a temporomandibular joint dislocation include yawning, undergoing dental work, and grinding or clenching the teeth.

Ⓟ Sore throats caused by a bacterium can progress to peritonsillar abscesses, retropharyngeal abscesses, rheumatic fever, and glomerulonephritis.

Ⓟ The symptoms of epiglottitis is usually less severe in adults then children.

Ⓟ Pinching the nostrils will NOT effectively control the bleeding of a posterior epistaxis because the bleeding site lies behind the cartilage of the nose.

Ⓟ The bleeding of a posterior epistaxis may be controlled by insertion of a nasal sponge or epistaxis balloon.

- Ⓟ Severe bleeding from the posterior nasopharynx may be controlled by inserting a 12 or 16 French urinary catheter into the affected nares and inflating the balloon.
- Ⓟ The tympanic membrane will appear normal on visualization with otitis externa because the infection affects only the outer ear canal, not the inner ear.
- Ⓟ Patients with Meniere's disease may have nystagmus and signs of vagal stimulation (abdominal pain, diaphoresis, bradycardia and pallor.)
- Ⓟ Flying insects will fly towards light, therefore, place the patient with a flying insect in the external ear in a darkened room and shine a light in the ear canal to draw the insect out.
- Ⓟ Non-flying insects (e.g. cockroaches and spiders) cannot back up, therefore, they must be removed by instilling mineral oil or 2% lidocaine jelly in the external ear canal, then flushing the dead insect out.

- ⓟ Loss of sensation to the lower lip indicates damage to the inferior alveolar nerve (often associated with mandibular fractures).
- ⓟ Patients with ocular entrapment may complain of diplopia.
- ⓟ Mandibular fractures cause pain, tenderness, edema and deformities to the lower face, excessive salivation, drooling and hematomas to the face and lower gum line.
- ⓟ The eighth cranial nerve is the acoustic nerve and is responsible for hearing and equilibrium.
- ⓟ Antiviral agents and steroids are used to decrease the symptoms associated with Bell's palsy.
- ⓟ Because of the proximity of the nerve to an Ellis class two fracture, patients will find the tooth sensitive to cold and heat. Calcium hydroxide paste is applied to protect the tooth.
- ⓟ Diuretics may be prescribed for patients with Meniere's disease to stabilize body fluids and reduce symptoms.

- ℗ Patients with temporomandibular joint dislocations may have difficulty maintaining an airway, suctioning may be required.
- ℗ White or yellow patches may be seen on the throat of a patient with a sore throat caused by a bacterium.
- ℗ Antibiotics are used to treat sore throats with a bacterial cause.
- ℗ The classic sign of epiglottitis is a high fever with a severe sore throat and drooling.
- ℗ Green exudate from the ear canal signifies otitis externa caused by gram-negative bacteria.
- ℗ Yellow, crusty exudate from the ear canal signifies an otitis externa caused by staphylococcus aureus.
- ℗ Fluffy white or black material growing out of the ear canal signifies an otitis externa caused by fungus.
- ℗ The pain of otitis media is usually worse when a patient lies prone.

Ⓟ Bacterial labrynthitis is treated with antibiotics, viral labrynthitis must run its course. Anti-emetics and anti-histamines would be prescribed for both diagnoses.

Ⓟ Children may not verbalize that they have a foreign body in the nose. The first sign may be a foul smell, redness, swelling and bleeding from one nostril.

Ⓟ Sinusitis of the frontal sinus causes pain over the forehead or around the orbit. The pain is exacerbated by leaning forward.

Ⓟ Sinusitis in the maxillary sinus causes pain below the eyes, over the cheekbones, upper teeth, or upper jaw, ear pain, pain with chewing, and numbness over middle third of face.

Ⓟ Sinusitis in the ethmoid sinus causes pain at the bridge of the nose, behind the eyes, and mastoid pain.

Ⓟ Sinusitis in the sphenoid sinus causes pain at the bridge of the nose, behind the eyes, and mastoid pain.

- ℗ Numbness of the upper lip is associated with maxillary fractures and damage to the infraorbital nerve.
- ℗ Patients who fall with sharp objects in their mouth may lacerate the hard or soft palate.
- ℗ Patients who present with neck trauma complicated by aphasia or hemiplegia may have damage to the large vessels of the neck causing decreased blood supply to the brain or spinal cord.
- ℗ A patient with Bell's palsy may demonstrate Bell's phenomenon, where the eye rolls up in the head when the patient attempts to close the affected eyelid.
- ℗ Patients with an Ellis class two tooth fracture should be instructed to see a dentist within 24 hours to have the tooth repaired and reduce the risk of infection.
- ℗ Patients being discharged with a sore throat should be encouraged to use antipyretics and analgesics as needed, and rinse the mouth and throat with warm saline gargles.

- Ⓟ Laryngitis is a viral infection that causes hoarseness.
- Ⓟ Epiglottitis causes a severe sore throat with redness and edema around the epiglottis.
- Ⓟ If the ear canal is severely swollen due to otitis externa, a small piece of gauze or other absorbent material (ear wick or otowick) may be inserted into the ear.
- Ⓟ When visualized, the tympanic membrane of a patient with otitis media will appear erythematous and dull and may appear to bulge.
- Ⓟ Sinusitis is treated with antibiotics.
- Ⓟ Signs of orbital fractures include facial numbness, subcutaneous emphysema of the face, eye pain, subconjunctival hemorrhages, enophthalmos or exophthalmos.
- Ⓟ An infection of the tonsils (tonsillitis) can spread into the tonsillar beds causing a condition known as a peritonsillar abscess.

- Ⓟ The respiratory distress associated with croup is usually less severe than epiglottitis.
- Ⓟ Otitis externa is treated with antibiotic-steroid ear drops.
- Ⓟ Meclizine (Antivert) is used to treat nausea for inner ear disorders.
- Ⓟ Lack of pupillary response may indicate damage to the oculomotor nerve.
- Ⓟ Hematomas of the ear should be drained to prevent development of a deformity known as a "cauliflower" ear.
- Ⓟ Peritonsillar abscesses carry a risk of airway obstruction.
- Ⓟ Epiglottitis may progress to complete airway obstruction.
- Ⓟ Treatment for otitis media includes antibiotics, adequate hydration, and analgesics.
- Ⓟ Antihistamines are prescribed for inner ear disorders to increase blood flow to the inner ear which minimizes vertigo.
- Ⓟ Vincent's angina is an infection of the gums and lining of the mouth.

Ⓟ Lack of appropriate eye movement through all the visual fields indicates injury to cranial nerves III, IV and VI or fractures of the orbit of the eye with entrapment of the ocular nerves and muscles.

Ⓟ Signs of esophageal trauma include dysphagia, hematemesis, chest pain, and odynophagia.

Ⓟ Symptoms of a peritonsillar abscess include a reddened, painful, and swollen pharynx. The patient may speak with a muffled tone and may have difficulty swallowing saliva.

Ⓟ Signs of epiglottitis include assumption of the tripod position, dysphasia, drooling, inspiratory stridor, expiratory snore, and retractions.

Ⓟ Steroids may be prescribed for inner ear disorders to reduce inflammation. Anticholinergics may be given to reduce vagal-mediated gastrointestinal symptoms.

Ⓟ Benzodiazepines are given to patients with inner ear disorders to sedate the vestibular system.

- Ⓟ The ninth cranial nerve is the glossopharyngeal nerve and is partially responsible for swallowing, the gag reflex, and the ability to taste on the posterior tongue.
- Ⓟ The pain of trigeminal neuralgia may be triggered by exposure to cold or facial stimulus such as eating, drinking, washing the face, shaving, applying make-up, or a light breeze to the face.
- Ⓟ Patient's with Bell's palsy will have sensation to the cornea on the affected side but may not blink if the cornea is stimulated.
- Ⓟ A patient with temporal arteritis may have systemic signs of infection such as night sweats, fever, and aching joints.
- Ⓟ Ludwig's angina causes the lower face to appear swollen and erythematous. The soft tissue of the lower face may be hard to the touch.
- Ⓟ An avulsed tooth is one which is no longer in its socket.
- Ⓟ Temporomandibular joint dislocations are reduced using procedural sedation.

- ℗ The pus of a peritonsillar abscess may be withdrawn with needle aspiration. Severe cases may require an incision and drainage of the tonsillar bed.
- ℗ The symptoms of croup often start with an upper respiratory tract infection that progress to the classic barky cough.
- ℗ Epiglottitis often has an abrupt onset.
- ℗ When discharging a patient with otitis externa, encourage them to avoid activities such as showering and swimming which would cause the external auditory meatus to become wet.
- ℗ To remove a foreign body from the nose, occlude the unaffected side and ask the patient to blow their nose.
- ℗ Lack of sensation to one side of the face can be indicative of damage to cranial nerve V.
- ℗ Anesthetics containing epinephrine should not be used to repair lacerations of the ear or nose, secondary to their vasoconstrictive properties.

Ⓟ Zygomatic and orbital fractures carry a high risk for cervical spinal and intracranial injuries.

Ⓟ The tenth cranial nerve is the vagus nerve and shares responsibility with the glossopharyngeal nerve for swallowing and gag reflex.

Ⓟ The pain of trigeminal neuralgia comes in waves that may only last for a few seconds but may reoccur many times throughout a day. Patients may have pain free intervals.

Ⓟ To prevent drying or ulceration of the cornea, patient's with Bell's palsy should be taught to instill lubricating eye drops. If the eye does not close at all, a patch may be applied.

Ⓟ Patients being discharged home after treatment of a peritonsillar abscess need to be taught how to rinse with half strength hydrogen peroxide and warmed saline.

Ⓟ The patient with a ruptured tympanic membrane should be reassured that the membrane will heal itself and the ear canal should be kept dry until healing is complete.

Ⓟ The cough and respiratory distress of croup is often more severe at night when the patient is less likely to swallow their secretions.

Ⓟ Causes of ruptured tympanic membranes include severe otitis media, barotraumas, or blast waves from explosions.

Ⓟ When a tympanic membrane ruptures, the patient may experience sudden severe pain followed by drainage of serous or serosanguinous fluid. The patient will often have decreased pain and hearing afterwards.

Ⓟ The eleventh cranial nerve is the spinal accessory nerve which allows head and shoulder movement.

Ⓟ Temporal arteritis carries the potential of causing decreased visual acuity or even blindness.

Ⓟ Patients with vertigo secondary to inner ear disorders should be encouraged to lie still with their eyes closed during the acute exacerbation.

- Ⓟ To test the zygomatic branch of cranial nerve seven, ask the patient close their eyes tightly. They will be unable to do so if the nerve is injured.
- Ⓟ To test the temporal branch of cranial nerve seven, ask the patient to elevate the brow or wrinkle the forehead. Inability to do so indicates injury to this nerve.
- Ⓟ To test the buccal branch of cranial nerve seven, ask the patient to elevate the upper lip, wrinkle the nose, or whistle. Inability to do any of these activities indicates the nerve is injured.
- Ⓟ Trauma to the thyroid gland may lead to thyroid storm.
- Ⓟ Patients with sinusitis should be discouraged from using nasal decongestants for more than 3—4 consecutive days to prevent mucosal rebound effect.
- Ⓟ Patients with mandibular fractures carry a risk of airway obstruction from edema, secretions, and instability of the anatomical structures responsible for swallowing.

- Ⓟ Elevate the head of the bed and apply ice to the face of a patient with an orbital or zygomatic fracture.
- Ⓟ To prevent exacerbation of their condition, patients with Bell's palsy should be instructed to avoid cold drafts to the face.
- Ⓟ The retropharyngeal space is an area that extends from the base of the skull to the mediastinum in the area around the nasopharynx, oropharynx, pharynx, and larynx.
- Ⓟ Treatment for croup includes administration of cool, humidified air or oxygen and adequate hydration. Racemic epinephrine may be prescribed for severe exacerbations.
- Ⓟ An infection in the retropharyngeal space is called a retropharyngeal abscess.
- Ⓟ For a child with epiglottitis, excess stimulation of the patient can cause spasms of the epiglottic folds leading to complete airway obstruction.

Ⓟ Patients being discharged after placement of an ear wick or otowick need to be taught to leave it in place until it falls out on its own.

Ⓟ Discharge instructions for patients diagnosed with Meniere's disease includes stressing the importance of fluid replenishment secondary to sweating.

Ⓟ Aside from facial swelling, additional symptoms of Ludwig's angina includes fever, chills, trismus, dysphagia, and dysphasia.

Ⓟ Causes of Vincent's angina include mouth breathing, emotional stressors, nutritional deficiencies, smoking, and upper respiratory tract infections.

Ⓟ Avulsed teeth should be re-implanted as quickly as possible to increase the chance of successful re-implantation. Re-implantation should occur within six hours of the avulsion.

Ⓟ When discharging a patient who has had a reduction of a temporomandibular joint dislocation, encourage them to avoid activities such as yawning and teeth clenching or grinding.

Ⓟ Potential complications of a retropharyngeal abscess include airway obstruction, erosion of the carotid artery, jugular venous thrombosis, epidural abscesses, and pneumonia.

Ⓟ Do not force interventions such as taking a temperature, or starting an intravenous line on a child with epiglottitis, if it will cause the child to cry or become upset.

Ⓟ An Ellis class three tooth fracture will cause the affected tooth to appear pink or blood-tinged.

Ⓟ Incision and drainage of the base of the mouth is used to decrease the edema of Ludwig's angina, followed by antibiotic administration.

Ⓟ Temporal arteritis is diagnosed with a biopsy of the affected blood vessel.

Ⓟ Patients with Vincent's angina will present with a foul smelling odor on their breath, and a gray pseudomembrane which lines the inside of the mouth and will bleed when removed.

- Ⓟ Cover an Ellis class three tooth fracture with dental foil or gauze for both patient comfort and to reduce the risk of infection.
- Ⓟ Provide analgesia to a patient with temporomandibular joint dislocations both before and after reduction. Encourage them to apply ice to the face for pain after discharge.
- Ⓟ Symptoms of a retropharyngeal abscess include a sore throat, neck stiffness, swelling, stridor, drooling, fever and, cervical lymphadenopathy.
- Ⓟ The pain of otitis externa may be diminished with application of heat to the eternal ear.
- Ⓟ If posterior packing is used to control a posterior epistaxis, monitor closely for an airway obstruction afterwards.
- Ⓟ To reduce vertigo, patients with inner ear disorders should be taught to limit activity, maintain bed rest, move slowly, and change positions slowly.
- Ⓟ Trigeminal neuralgia is a form of neurogenic pain.

Ⓟ Handle an avulsed tooth by the crown, never touching the exposed ligaments and nerves.

Ⓟ Ⓟ To remove a foreign object from a nostril, a urinary catheter may be placed in the nose, the balloon inflated, then the urinary catheter withdrawn.

Ⓟ Temporal arteritis is diagnosed with a biopsy of the affected blood vessel.

Ⓟ Cover an Ellis class three tooth fracture with dental foil or gauze for both patient comfort and to reduce the risk of infection.

Ⓟ Provide analgesia to a patient with temporomandibular joint dislocations both before and after reduction. Encourage them to apply ice to the face for pain after discharge.

Ⓟ Symptoms of a retropharyngeal abscess include a sore throat, neck stiffness, swelling, stridor, drooling, fever and, cervical lymphadenopathy.

Ⓟ The pain of otitis externa may be diminished with application of heat to the eternal ear.

Ⓟ If posterior packing is used to control a posterior epistaxis, monitor closely for an airway obstruction afterwards.

Ⓟ To reduce vertigo, patients with inner ear disorders should be taught to limit activity, maintain bed rest, move slowly, and change positions slowly.

Ⓟ Patients with epiglottitis will often be intubated either in the emergency department or the operating room. Surgical airways may sometimes be required due to swelling of the airway.

Ⓟ Patients with sinusitis should be encouraged to rest with the upper body elevated to facilitate drainage of the sinuses.

Ⓟ Trauma to the brachial plexus causes pain in the neck and shoulder, paresthesias of an upper limb, or weakness and heaviness in an upper extremity.

- Ⓟ Patients with LeFort fractures are often unable to maintain their own airway and will require frequent suctioning, intubation, or a surgical airway.
- Ⓟ Encourage patients with orbital and zygomatic fractures to avoid activities such as Valsalva's maneuver, straining, or blowing the nose to prevent the development of subcutaneous emphysema.
- Ⓟ Temporal arteritis is treated with steroids and analgesics.
- Ⓟ Patients with mandibular fractures should be cared for in the high Fowler's position when possible.
- Ⓟ The twelfth cranial nerve is the hypoglossal nerve and is responsible for movement of the tongue.
- Ⓟ Treatment for trigeminal neuralgia may include anti-convulsants and anti-depressants. In severe cases, surgery may be required.
- Ⓟ Warm packs to the face and facial massage may decrease the discomfort associated with Bell's palsy.

- Ⓟ Patients with Ludwig's angina should be taught how to rinse with half strength hydrogen peroxide rinses and to apply ice to the area after incision and drainage.
- Ⓟ Treatment for Vincent's angina includes local debridement, mouth care with half-strength hydrogen peroxide rinses, and antibiotics.
- Ⓟ Ellis class three tooth fractures constitute a dental emergency and immediate referral to a dentist should be facilitated.
- Ⓟ While awaiting re-implantation, an avulsed teeth may be preserved placing it in a glass of Hank's balanced electrolyte solution (preferred), or in a glass of milk or saline.
- Ⓟ Discharge teaching for a patient who has undergone a temporo-mandibular joint reduction includes the consumption of a soft diet for 3 – 4 days to reduce chewing motion.
- Ⓟ Treatment of a retropharyngeal abscess includes antibiotics as well as incision and drainage of the infection, sometimes in the operating room.

- Ⓟ A complete blood count, coagulation studies, and a type and cross-match is typically drawn on patients who present with significant epistaxis.
- Ⓟ Patients with otitis externa need to be discouraged from using cotton tipped applicators in their ears until the infection has completely resolved.
- Ⓟ Once the airway of a patient with epiglottitis is secured, antibiotics are used to treat the infection.
- Ⓟ Substances which can exacerbate symptoms of Meniere's disease include salt and sugar intake, caffeine, alcohol, and smoking.
- Ⓟ 1% phenylephrine may be applied topically to reduce swelling prior to attempting removal of a foreign object from the nostril.
- Ⓟ Wrap avulsed parts of the face in sterile gauze moistened with normal saline, place in a plastic bag, and then place in a basin filled with normal saline and ice .
- Ⓟ Apply ice to the lower face of a patient with a mandibular fracture.

Ⓟ Apply ice to the face of a patient with LeFort fractures.

Ⓟ Cerebrospinal fluid tastes sweet. The patient with a head injury that describes a sweet tasting post-nasal drip should be assessed for possible basilar skull fractures.

Ⓟ Priorities of care for patients with neck trauma include maintenance of a patent airway, cervical spinal precautions, adequate oxygenation, control of blood loss, and frequent neurological assessments.

Ⓟ Heat to the face may relieve pressure and pain associated with sinusitis.

Ⓟ Because trigeminal neuralgia is a neuropathic pain, it responds to adjuvant analgesics such as carbamazepine (Tegretol), Phenytoin (Dilantin), Oxcarbazepine (Trileptal), Clonazepam (Klonopin), Lamotrigine (Lamictal), Valproic acid (Depakene) or Gabapentin (Neurontin)

- ℗ Ocular entrapment causes the eye to be locked in the downward and outward position with pain when the patient attempts to look upwards.
- ℗ Entrapment of the infraorbital nerve, often associated with a fracture of the zygomatic bone, will cause numbness to the cheek, lower eyelid and upper lip on the same side as the injury.
- ℗ Encourage patients to warm ear drops prior to instillation. Cold drops may cause dizziness, warm drops decrease this possibility.
- ℗ Mastoiditis is an infection of the mastoid bone that is often related to untreated ear infections. With antibiotic therapy, this condition is uncommon today.
- ℗ Untreated mastoiditis may lead to meningitis and encephalitis.
- ℗ Symptoms of labrynthitis include vertigo (associated with movement), hearing loss, tinnitus, nausea and vomiting, nystagmus and fever.

- Ⓟ Encourage patients with symptoms of dizziness to lie still with the eyes closed during episodes of dizziness to reduce the risk of injury.
- Ⓟ Treatment for labrynthitis includes encouraging bed rest and adequate hydration. Pharmacological interventions may include antiemetics, benzodiazepines, oral corticosteroids and antibiotics.
- Ⓟ Button batteries in body orifices continue to conduct electrical impulses and can cause significant tissue necrosis. Therefore, they should be removed expeditiously.

Bibliography for maxillofacial emergencies

Amsterdam, J. T. (2014). Oral Medicine. In J. A. Marx, R. S. Hockberger, & R. M. Walls, *Rosen's Emergency Medicine* (pp. 895 - 908). Philadelphia: Elsevier.

Andreoni, C. (2013). Pediatric Considerations in Emergency Nursing. In B. B. Hammond, & P. Gerber-Zimmerman (Eds.), *Sheehy's Emergency Nursing: Principals and Practice* (7 ed., pp. 547 - 570). Philadelphia: Elsevier.

Asensio, J. A., & Trunkey, D. D. (2016). Initital Assessment and Resuscitation. In *Therapy of Trauma and Surgical Critical Care* (2 ed., pp. 57 - 69). Philadelphia: Elsevier.

Bhatia, K., & Sharma, R. (2013). Eye Emergencies. In J. G. Adams, *Emergency Medicine* (pp. 209 - 225). Philadelphia: Elsevier.

Centers for Disease Control and Prevention. (2014, January 9). *Conjunctivitis (Pink Eye)*. Retrieved from Centers for Disease Control and Prevention: http://www.cdc.gov/conjunctivitis/clinical.html

Chi, J. J., & Alam, D. S. (2014). Facial Trauma. In J. L. Cameron, & A. M. Cameron, *Current Surgical Therapy* (11 ed., pp. 1070 - 1081). Philadelphia: Elsevier.

Dahl, A. A. (2015, May 14). *Keratitis*. Retrieved from MedicineNet.com: http://www.medicinenet.com/keratitis/article.htm

Egging, D. (2013). Facial, ENT, and Dental Emergencies. In B. B. Hammond, & P. Gerber-Zimmerman (Eds.), *Sheehy's Emergency Nursing: Principals and Practice* (7 ed., pp. 275 - 289). Philadelphia: Elsevier.

Mays, M., Kabongo, M. L., & Satya-Murti, S. (January 31, 2012). *Trigeminal Neuralgia*. Retrieved from First Consult: https://www.clinicalkey.com/#!/content/medical_topic/21-s2.0-1014499

Misulis, K. E., Galloway, G. M., & Harper, W. (2010, August 10). *Bell's Palsy*. Retrieved from First Consult: https://www.clinicalkey.com/#!/content/medical_topic/21-s2.0-1014441

Muchatuta, M. N. (2015, December 14). *Iritis and Uveitis*. Retrieved from MedScape: http://emedicine.medscape.com/article/798323-overview

National Institutes of Health. (2010, July). *Meniere's Disease*. Retrieved from National Institute on Deafness and Other Communication Disorders: http://www.nidcd.nih.gov/health/balance/pages/meniere.aspx

Peng, L. F. (2014, December 31). *Avulsed Tooth Treatment and Management*. Retrieved from MedScape: http://emedicine.medscape.com/article/763291-treatment

Watkins, T. A., Opie , N. J., & Norman, A. (2011, August 1). Airway choices in maxillofacial trauma. *Trends in Anesthesia and Critical Care, 1*(4), 179 – 190

NEUROLOGICAL
EMERGENCIES

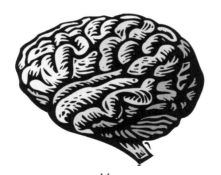

Ⓟ Fungal meningitis is usually found in patients with pre-existing immunocompromise.

Ⓟ Viral meningitis is often mild, short-lived and non-contagious.

Ⓟ Brain injured patients tend to lose orientation to event first, followed by loss of orientation to time next, then place and person is usually the last sphere of orientation to be lost.

Ⓟ Intracranial pressure below 10 mm Hg is considered normal, when pressures reach 15 mm Hg they are considered elevated. Pressures above 20 mm Hg are called intracranial hypertension.

Ⓟ The most mobile parts of the spinal cord are the cervical spine and the thoracic spine at the level of T11 and T12. Therefore, these are the areas most likely be injured in spinal cord injury.

Ⓟ Pain below the level of a spinal cord injury can result in autonomic dysreflexia. Possible causes of autonomic dysreflexia include urinary retention, constipation, renal colic, decubitus ulcers and appendicitis.

- Ⓟ Examples of primary headaches include migraine headaches, cluster headaches and tension headaches.
- Ⓟ A secondary headache is one which is caused by something else. Treatment for a secondary headache involves treating the underlying cause.
- Ⓟ Dementia is defined as a global deterioration of cognitive function in two or more areas without impaired consciousness.
- Ⓟ If the entire brain seizes, it is called a generalized seizure; if only part of the brain seizes it is called a partial seizure.
- Ⓟ Because nerves cross over in the spinal cord, weakness on one side of the body indicates damage or injury to the opposite side of the brain.
- Ⓟ To assess motor function in the responsive patient, ask them to perform a task that allows assessment of both sides of the body, such as squeezing fingers. This allows assessment for lateralization.

- ℗ Lateralization is loss of strength on one side of the body when compared with the other side.
- ℗ Epidural bleeds are usually arterial, therefore the patient's condition will decline rapidly and mortality is high.
- ℗ Early signs of increased intracranial pressure include anxiety, restlessness, loss of orientation, memory alterations and increasing stimulation to elicit a patient response as time passes.
- ℗ A late sign of increased intracranial pressure (often associated with herniation of the brain) is a depressed level of consciousness. The patient may respond only to deep pain or be completely unarousable.
- ℗ Indications of an obstructed CSF shunt include signs of increasing intracranial pressure such as irritability, headache, neck pain, vomiting, and bulging fontanels.
- ℗ A partial spinal cord syndrome is one in which some sensory or motor function is preserved below the injury.

Ⓟ Patients with epidural bleeds may have a history of unconsciousness at the time of injury followed by a period of lucidity, then another rapid decline in the level of consciousness.

Ⓟ A complete spinal cord syndrome is one in which there is no preservation of motor or sensory function below the injury.

Ⓟ Bacterial meningitis is serious and contagious. It may lead to increased intracranial pressure and death within hours of onset in severe cases.

Ⓟ Diffuse axonal injuries and concussions are considered diffuse brain injuries that affect a large, rather than localized area of the brain.

Ⓟ Causes of dementia include Alzheimer's disease (most common), vascular changes, infections, inflammatory changes, neoplasms ,trauma, metabolic alterations, and hydrocephalic changes.

Ⓟ Risk factors for dementia include aging, smoking, hypercholesterolemia, obesity, diabetes, genetics (especially Alzheimer's) and Parkinson's disease.

- ℗ Headaches, nausea and vomiting are the most common early symptoms of intracranial bleeds and hemorrhagic strokes.
- ℗ Guillain Barré syndrome usually starts with tingling in the lower extremities that begins several weeks after a viral illness.
- ℗ There are three stages to a tonic-clonic seizure: tonic phase, clonic phase and post-ictal phase.
- ℗ Sources of bacterial meningitis include blood-borne infections, basilar skull fractures, infected facial structures, and brain abscesses.
- ℗ Infection in a CSF drainage shunt is most likely to occur within a few months of placement and may cause obstruction, local wound problems or unexplained fevers.
- ℗ To assess pronator drift, ask patients to close their eyes, hold their hands directly in front of them with the palms up for 30 seconds and look for one arm to drift down before the other.
- ℗ The suffix for weakness is "-paresis" and the suffix for paralysis is "-plegia".

Ⓟ To test motor function in the unresponsive patient, apply noxious stimuli, such as pinching the trapezius muscle or pushing on the patient's nail beds.

Ⓟ In early increasing intracranial pressure, the pupils may be sluggish to respond to light, in late increased intracranial pressure, they may be fixed and/or dilated.

Ⓟ A communicating depressed skull fracture may cause seizures.

Ⓟ Uncomplicated linear skull fractures may be discharged home.

Ⓟ Indications of an epidural bleed include severe headaches and indications of rapidly increasing intracranial pressures.

Ⓟ Patients with spinal cord injuries above the level of C4 will lose use of all respiratory muscles and will have complete respiratory paralysis.

Ⓟ Migraine headaches typically cause severe, pulsatile, throbbing pain to one side of the head.

Ⓟ A subarachnoid hemorrhage is often caused by the rupture of an aneurysm in the subarachnoid space. It may also be caused by trauma to the head.

Ⓟ The use of hyperventilation to treat intracranial pressure is reserved for patients who have signs of cranial herniation for which other interventions have been ineffective.

Ⓟ Indications of dementia include memory loss, noticeable personality changes, disorientation, repetitive speech and disorientation.

Ⓟ Cluster headaches tend to cause unilateral severe, burning, sharp, excruciating pain in the periorbital or temporal regions of the head.

Ⓟ Increased intracranial pressure due to meningitis may cause headaches (especially occipital), vomiting, anorexia, altered mental status, hyperreflexia and seizures.

Ⓟ Sensory deficits related to a stroke tend to start on one side of the face and progress to the arm and finally the leg.

- ℗ Patients with dementia often exhibit sundowning (symptoms get worse as the day progresses).
- ℗ Symptoms of Guillain Barré include an ascending symmetrical paralysis with associated loss of deep tendon reflexes.
- ℗ The tonic phase of a tonic-clonic seizure is marked by dilated pupils, incontinence and stiff extension of the arms and legs.
- ℗ When noxious stimuli is applied to an unresponsive patient and they reach for the stimuli, it is termed "localization to pain".
- ℗ Infants with bacterial meningitis may demonstrate poor feeding, headache, high-pitched cry, bulging of the fontanelles, hyperreflexia and seizures.
- ℗ When an unresponsive patient pulls away from the application of noxious stimuli, it is termed "withdrawal from pain".
- ℗ In early increasing intracranial pressure, the patient may have weakness contra-lateral to the lesion, in late increased intracranial pressure, they may exhibit dense hemiparesis, or abnormal flexion or extension.

- Ⓟ Patients with spinal cord injuries between C5 and T1 will have respiratory insufficiency and may require intubation and respiratory support during the acute phase of the injury.
- Ⓟ Visual changes associated with a stroke include diplopia, loss of visual fields and amaurosis fugax (a visual alteration where the patient describes a gray shade slowly pulled over one eye).
- Ⓟ Ruptures of subarachnoid aneurysms typically occur between the fifth and sixth decade of life.
- Ⓟ Patients with dementia are unaware of their cognitive deterioration
- Ⓟ The paralysis of Guillain Barré may ascend only partially in some patients, in others, it may ascend all the way to the head, leading to complete body paralysis.
- Ⓟ Dementia is non-reversible cognitive changes, delirium is reversible cognitive changes.
- Ⓟ A position of abnormal flexion is also known as decorticate posturing.

Ⓟ Anterior circulation strokes typically cause weakness.

Ⓟ The clonic phase of a tonic-clonic seizure is marked by strenuous, rhythmic muscle contractions with hyperventilation, profuse sweating, tachycardia and excessive salivation.

Ⓟ Decorticate posturing (flexion posture) is flexion and adduction of the arms, wrists and fingers while the legs are fully extended and internally rotated. The feet are plantar flexed.

Ⓟ Pupillary changes are ipsilateral to brain lesions, motor function changes are generally contralateral to the lesion.

Ⓟ Mannitol (Osmitrol, Resectisol) is an osmotic diuretic that can quickly reduce intracranial pressure but can lead to fluid and electrolyte imbalances and pulmonary edema.

Ⓟ Treatment for epidural bleeding includes skull trephination or surgical decompression of the hematoma as well as interventions to decrease intracranial pressure.

Ⓟ Vertigo is associated with posterior circulation strokes.

- Ⓟ The arms are innervated between C5 and T1, therefore injuries in this area will result in loss of arm movement and sensation. The higher the injury, the more severe the deficit.
- Ⓟ Autonomic dysreflexia results in sympathetic stimulation below the level of the spinal cord injury and parasympathetic stimulation above the level of the injury.
- Ⓟ The infectious processes of meningitis may cause symptoms such as fever, chills, malaise, weakness, and elevated temperature (infants and elderly may be hypothermic).
- Ⓟ Tests which may reveal the causes of delirium include serum chemistries, vitamin B_{12} levels, testing for syphilis, Lyme disease and HIV, thyroid function tests and toxicology levels.
- Ⓟ Depressed skull fractures and basilar skull fractures carry a high rate of meningitis.
- Ⓟ Patients with spinal cord injuries below the level of T1 will usually be able to breathe spontaneously.

Ⓟ Communication changes associated with a stroke include dysarthria (slurred speech), expressive aphasia (cannot use words appropriately), and receptive aphasia (cannot understand words).

Ⓟ A concussion results in a temporary loss of consciousness with amnesia surrounding the event.

Ⓟ Spinal cord injuries between L1 and L4 will result in loss of ability to extend and flex the legs.

Ⓟ Spinal cord injuries between L5 and S4 will cause loss of ability to flex the foot and extend the toes.

Ⓟ The post-ictal phase of a tonic-clonic seizure is marked by a depressed level of consciousness, confusion, deep breathing, headache, muscle aches, and fatigue.

Ⓟ Patients with a CSF drainage shunt that ends in the abdomen are at risk for developing peritonitis.

Ⓟ Absence seizures are most common in children between the ages of 4 and 12.

- ℗ The pain of a tension headache is usually described as dull and non-pulsating. It starts in the occiput, moves bilaterally to the front of the scalp around the hatband area of the skull.
- ℗ A position of abnormal extension is also known as decerebrate posturing.
- ℗ Decerebrate posturing is stiff extension of the arms while the legs are fully extended and internally rotated. The feet will be plantar flexed.
- ℗ To prevent severe fluid and electrolyte imbalances, the very young and old may be given loop or thiazide diuretics instead of Mannitol (Osmitrol, Resectisol) for increased ICP.
- ℗ Decorticate posturing is associated with lesions above the midbrain and decerebrate posturing is associated with an insult to the brainstem.
- ℗ Two risk factors for a subarachnoid bleed include old age and alcoholism.

- Ⓟ In a communicating depressed skull fracture, bone fragments contact cerebral tissue; in non-communicating depressed skull fractures, there is no cerebral contact.
- Ⓟ An absence seizure involves cessation of activity with loss of consciousness, usually for less than 15 seconds, but does not involve generalized clonic muscular movements.
- Ⓟ Children who require CSF drainage shunts as infants to drain CSF fluid may end up with excessive CSF drainage as they age. This is especially common as they learn to walk and are upright for longer periods.
- Ⓟ Motor function in response to painful stimuli degenerates in the following order: localization, withdrawal, decorticate posturing, decerebrate posturing and flaccidity.
- Ⓟ Signs of a concussion include nausea, vomiting, temporary amnesia, headaches and occasionally, a brief loss of vision.

- ℗ Meningitis caused by the bacteria *Neisseria meningitidis* is commonly known as meningococcal meningitis.
- ℗ Steroids are sometimes given to patients with increased intracranial pressure to reduce cerebral edema. This treatment can increase the risk of infection in the patient.
- ℗ When testing deep tendon reflexes, compare both limbs for symmetrical reaction.
- ℗ Patients with anterior cord syndromes will have loss of motor function below the level of the injury but retain some of their sensory function.
- ℗ Cranial nerve dysfunction associated with a stroke is ipsilateral to the affected side of the brain whereas muscle weakness or hemiplegia and loss of deep tendon reflexes will be contralateral to the affected side.
- ℗ Subarachnoid bleeds that become symptomatic within 48 hours are called acute subarachnoid bleeds.

- ℗ Patients with dementia and delirium need to be cared for in low stimulation environments. Leave the lights on in the room when possible to help the patient remain oriented.
- ℗ Cognitive function is unaffected with Guillain Barré syndrome.
- ℗ Symptoms of an anterior basilar skull fracture include anosmia, epistaxis, rhinorrhea, and loss of sensation to forehead, cornea and nose.
- ℗ Other symptoms of an anterior basilar skull fracture include subconjunctival hemorrhage, hemorrhage in the periorbital spaces (Racoon's eyes), visual disturbances, altered eye movement and ptosis.
- ℗ Migraine headaches usually last 4 to 72 hours.
- ℗ The usual length of a cluster headache is 15 to 180 minutes.
- ℗ Tension headaches may last as long as 7 days.
- ℗ Restraining a patient with dementia can increase confusion, disorientation, and general agitation.

ⓟ Meningitis caused by *Neisseria meningitidis* may result in a non-blanching petechial rash with spots 1 -2 millimeters in diameter on the trunk and lower portions of the body.

ⓟ Repetitive movements such as smacking the lips or twitching of the face, known as automatism, may be noted in patients having an absence seizure.

ⓟ The usual sites for deep tendon reflex testing are the Achilles tendon (ankle), the quadriceps (knee), the biceps and triceps (arm).

ⓟ Symptoms of a middle fossa basilar skull fracture include loss of sensation to lower face, otorrhea, deafness, tinnitus, facial palsy, and hemotympanum.

ⓟ Hypotonic solutions may worsen intracranial pressure in brain injured patients. Isotonic or hypertonic solutions will be chosen instead.

ⓟ Symptoms of a posterior fossa basilar skull fracture include ecchymosis behind the ear (battle sign), and impaired gag reflex.

- ℗ If it takes more than 48 hours but less than 14 days after an injury for a subarachnoid bleed to become symptomatic, it is called a subacute subarachnoid bleed.
- ℗ Slow bleeding blood vessels in the subarachnoid space may take more than 14 days to cause symptoms. This is called a chronic subarachnoid bleed.
- ℗ The symptoms of a subarachnoid bleed are similar to an epidural bleed, except they take longer to manifest.
- ℗ Nuchal rigidity, one sign of meningitis, is an inability to flex the neck forward due to rigidity of neck muscles.
- ℗ Patients with posterior cord syndromes will have loss of sensation but may retain some or all motor function below the level of the injury.
- ℗ Patients with central cord syndromes will lose motor and sensory function to the upper body but retain that function to the lower part of the body.

- Ⓟ Movement and activity tends to aggravate the pain of a migraine headache.
- Ⓟ Aneurysm ruptures are often precipitated by activities such as performing Valsalva's maneuver, bending forward, sneezing, coughing and other activities that increase intracranial pressure.
- Ⓟ Common symptoms of a stroke include gait abnormalities, hypertension, unilateral pronator drift, and nystagmus.
- Ⓟ There is no treatment for Guillain Barré syndrome. Respiratory weakness associated with the disorder may require mechanical ventilation. Physical therapy to maintain muscle mass during paralysis will be provided.
- Ⓟ Status epilepticus is either a series of consecutive seizures or a single seizure that does not respond to treatment.
- Ⓟ To test the corneal reflex, brush a wisp of cotton against the cornea or apply a small drop of water or saline to the cornea. The eye should rapidly close.

℗ The corneal, gag and swallow reflex are normal when present and abnormal when absent.

℗ The head of the bed should be elevated 15 to 30 degrees to reduce intracranial pressure in brain injured patients.

℗ Patients with autonomic dysreflexia will have flushing above the level of the spinal cord injury and coolness below the level of the injury.

℗ To elicit Kernig's sign, a possible indication of meningitis, bend the patient's leg at the hip and knee and then straighten it out. Pain or resistance on stretching out the leg is a positive sign.

℗ To elicit Brudzinski's sign, a possible indication of meningitis, bend a patient's neck forward. If the knees and hips flex, this is a positive sign.

℗ Reorient demented patients with repetitive statements as required.

℗ To test the gag reflex, stimulate the back of the pharynx. The patient should retch or gag.

Ⓟ To test the swallowing reflex, touch the patient's uvula, it should elevate.

Ⓟ Every effort to maintain the head of a brain injured patient midline should be undertaken to maximize venous drainage from subclavian vessels.

Ⓟ Discharge instructions for concussion include monitoring for changes in levels of consciousness, onset of projectile vomiting, unequal pupils, and increasing confusion.

Ⓟ Linear fractures which cross major blood vessels such as the middle meningeal artery carry a higher risk of intracranial bleeding.

Ⓟ Symptoms of autonomic dysreflexia include severe head headache, nasal stuffiness, patient anxiety, increased intracranial pressure, hypertension, sweating, and cardiac dysrhythmias.

Ⓟ Brown-Séquard syndrome is commonly associated with penetrating trauma, tumors or hematomas which affect one side of the spinal cord.

- Ⓟ Brown-Séquard syndrome causes loss of motor function to one side of the body, but retention of sensation to that side, yet loss of sensation to the other side with unaffected movement.
- Ⓟ Infants with meningitis may cry when held and settle when laid on a flat surface. This is termed paroxysmal irritability.
- Ⓟ To position infants, young children, obese patients or patients with bony deformities of the back for a lumbar puncture, use a sitting position with head and arms resting over a bedside table.
- Ⓟ A transient ischemic attack is a neurological deficit that resolves without treatment.
- Ⓟ Amyotrophic Lateral Sclerosis (ALS) is more commonly known as Lou Gehrig's disease.
- Ⓟ An odd sensation or sensory perception that occurs before the onset of a migraine headache is referred to as an aura.
- Ⓟ 30% of patients experience auras before the onset of a migraine headache.

- ℗ Cauda-equina syndrome causes varying degrees of motor and sensory function loss to the lower body, as well as problems with bowel and bladder control and alteration in sexual function.
- ℗ When using the sitting position for lumbar punctures, monitor for an occluded airway throughout the procedure.
- ℗ Cluster headaches tend to occur in clusters, typically 1 to 8 headaches per day lasting 60 to 90 minutes, often after falling asleep.
- ℗ The National Institute of Health Stroke Scale (NIHSS) is an objective score used to measure stroke severity, determine suitability for fibrinolytics, and establish inclusion/exclusion from clinical trials for stroke.
- ℗ The National Institute of Health Stroke Scale (NIHSS) should be administered by trained practitioners in a fairly rapid manner without any patient coaching.
- ℗ Plasmapheresis with immunoglobulin therapy may be considered early in Guillain Barré syndrome to decrease the severity of the symptoms.

Ⓟ Amyotrophic Lateral Sclerosis is a neurodegenerative disorder resulting in inability of voluntary motor nerves to transmit impulses causing loss of motor function and muscle degeneration.

Ⓟ Status epilepticus will result in acidosis, hypoglycemia, hypercalcemia, muscle damage, elevations in temperature, blood pressure and pulse and ultimately cerebral hypoxia with irreversible brain damage.

Ⓟ Symptoms of excessive drainage of a CSF drainage shunt include depressed fontanels or headaches that are worse when upright and improve when supine.

Ⓟ Partial seizures result in erratic and excessive electrical activity that affects only part of the brain.

Ⓟ The grasp reflex is normal in infancy but abnormal in adulthood. It is elicited by stimulating the inside of an unresponsive patient's hand. If the patient closes his or her fingers, it is an abnormal finding.

Ⓟ The Babinski reflex is normal in infancy but abnormal after a patient learns to walk. Stroke the lateral aspect of the foot, extension of the great toe is an abnormal finding.

Ⓟ Return of the grasp or Babinski reflex in adulthood is associated with severe neurological dysfunction.

Ⓟ Do not flex the hips of patients with increased intracranial pressure as this may further increase the pressure.

Ⓟ Meningeal fluid associated with bacterial meningitis appears cloudy with a white blood cell count of 2000 – 20,000/mm^{3}, low glucose levels, high protein levels and positive for bacteria.

Ⓟ Meningeal fluid associated with viral meningitis appears clear, with a white blood cell count less than 500/mm^{3}, normal glucose and protein levels and negative for bacteria.

Ⓟ The pupils of the eyes are normally no more than one millimeter different in size.

Ⓟ Central cord syndromes are more common in the elderly.

Ⓟ Non-narcotic rather than narcotic analgesia should be used to treat pain and headaches associated with concussions to prevent masking changes in level of consciousness.

Ⓟ The treatment for a subarachnoid bleed includes either skull trephination or surgical intervention as well as efforts to reduce intracranial pressure.

Ⓟ Sacral sparing is the retention of rectal tone and movement of the great toe. It is indicative of a partial cord syndrome.

Ⓟ Neurogenic shock is associated with spinal cord injuries above T4 to T6.

Ⓟ Men get tension headaches more commonly than women.

Ⓟ Symptoms which accompany the pain of a migraine include photophobia, phonophobia, facial paleness, nausea and vomiting.

Ⓟ Aniscoria is a difference of more than one millimeter between the pupils of the eyes and may be an indication of increased intracranial pressure.

- ℗ Elevated temperatures increase cerebral blood flow contributing to increased intracranial pressure. Therefore antipyretics and cooling blankets should be used to reduce temperatures in brain injured patients.
- ℗ Pupils which are irregularly or oval shaped may indicate increased intracranial pressure.
- ℗ Spinal shock usually occurs immediately after a spinal cord injury although it may appear as long as several days later.
- ℗ Reaction of the pupils to light may be described as brisk, sluggish, or nonreactive and fixed.
- ℗ Epi- means above and sub- means below. An epidural bleed is above the dura mater. A subarachnoid bleed is below the arachnoid mater, etc.
- ℗ Initiate droplet precautions when caring for a patient who may have bacterial meningitis.

Ⓟ Aniscoria coupled with diminished or absent reactivity of the pupils is a strong indicator of increased intracranial pressure.

Ⓟ Spinal shock is caused by a concussion to spinal cord tissue resulting in temporary loss of function of the nervous tissue.

Ⓟ Patients with cluster headaches often present with tearing, lid edema and eye redness to one side of the face as well as nasal congestion, sweating and pallor.

Ⓟ The National Institute of Health Stroke Scale (NIHSS) is scored based on how a patient responds, not how the practitioner feels the patient will respond.

Ⓟ A patient with a completely normal neurological exam and normal mental status will score 0 on the National Institute of Health Stroke Scale (NIHSS). This is a good score.

Ⓟ When bacterial meningitis is suspected, a lumbar puncture should be performed and intravenous antibiotics started immediately afterwards.

- Ⓟ When light is shone into the eye, it should constrict and the opposite pupil should simultaneously constrict (consensual reaction).
- Ⓟ Vital signs associated with increased intracranial pressure include elevated temperature, bradycardia, widened pulse pressure and abnormal respiratory patterns.
- Ⓟ Symptoms of post-concussion syndrome include headaches, positional dizziness, tinnitus, transient diplopia, inability to concentrate, memory disturbances and personality changes.
- Ⓟ Symptoms of post-concussion syndrome may last from several days to months or years after the concussion.
- Ⓟ Signs of spinal shock include flaccid paralysis, loss of reflexes and loss of bowel and bladder function.
- Ⓟ Treatment for meningitis is usually symptomatic, including antipyretics, analgesics and efforts to reduce intracranial pressure as needed.
- Ⓟ Rifampin (Rifadin) can permanently stain contact lenses.

Ⓟ The manifestations of spinal shock are temporary and will resolve. They may persist for a period of minutes or last several days or weeks.

Ⓟ Factors known to cause migraine headaches include sleep pattern changes, physical exertion, sudden changes in barometric pressure, stress, dieting, heat, lights, and cyclic estrogen levels.

Ⓟ The higher the National Institute of Health Stroke Scale (NIHSS) score, the worse the neurological damage the stroke has caused.

Ⓟ Indications of a subarachnoid bleed include severe head pain, nausea, vomiting, photophobia, phonophobia, sudden onset of seizures, nuchal rigidity and fevers.

Ⓟ A score of 15 – 20 using the National Institute of Health Stroke Scale (NIHSS) is considered a severe stroke.

Ⓟ Patients with indications of a stroke should be sent for a computerized tomography as soon after arrival as possible.

- Ⓟ The symptoms of a partial seizure may include automatism, twitching of one arm, or spastic contractions of the neck.
- Ⓟ Amyotrophic Lateral Sclerosis usually starts with twitching, cramping and stiffness in one limb that ultimately spreads to other muscles throughout the body.
- Ⓟ The majority of patients with Guillain Barré syndrome will experience a resolution of symptoms within a period of weeks to months.
- Ⓟ Manifestations of Amyotrophic Lateral Sclerosis include instability while walking and difficulty with fine motor control, such as doing up buttons or writing.
- Ⓟ Late Amyotrophic Lateral Sclerosis causes the respiratory and throat muscles to weaken leading to respiratory complications, choking and aspiration.
- Ⓟ Bradycardia is a late indicator of increased intracranial pressure.

- ℗ Pressure on the medulla in severely increased intracranial pressure may cause dysrhythmias including premature ventricular contractions, atrioventricular blocks and even ventricular fibrillation.
- ℗ Cheyne-stoke respirations are described as rhythmic crescendo and decresendo of rate and depth of respiration, interspersed with brief periods of apnea.
- ℗ Seizure activity can increase intracranial pressure.
- ℗ Symptoms of a diffuse axonal injury include altered levels of consciousness with abnormal posturing, hypertension, hyperthermia, and excessive sweating.
- ℗ The speech of a patient with Amyotrophic Lateral Sclerosis is often slurred and nasal.
- ℗ Sensory alterations in a partial seizure may include tingling or numbness to one part of the body or disturbances in sight, hearing, smell or taste.

- ℗ Central neurogenic hyperventilation is described as very deep and rapid respirations with no apneic periods.
- ℗ Apneustic breathing is described as prolonged inspiratory and/or expiratory pause of 2 – 3 seconds.
- ℗ Over drainage of a CSF drainage shunt puts a patient at risk for developing a subdural hematoma.
- ℗ All persons having close personal contact with a patient who is confirmed to have bacterial meningitis should receive prophylactic antibiotics.
- ℗ Neurogenic shock is the loss of sympathetic tone associated with spinal cord injury, spinal shock is temporary loss of function due to trauma to the spinal tissue.
- ℗ Minimizing movement will reduce intracranial pressure therefore medications such as propofol (Diprivan) and barbiturates are often administered to induce coma in brain injured patients.

- ℗ Patients with spinal cord injuries who hold their heads rigidly angulated or are unable to move their heads after the incident should be immobilized in the position found.
- ℗ Foods known to trigger migraine headaches include alcohol, caffeine, monosodium glutamate, ripened cheeses and coffee.
- ℗ A patient with complete hemiparesis, hemianopia, hemineglect, and aphasia would score 31 using the National Institute of Health Stroke Scale (NIHSS). This is the highest score possible on this scale.
- ℗ The CT scan of a patient with a diffuse axonal injury will be normal in the early stages.
- ℗ Ataxic respirations are described as irregular with random patterns of deep and shallow respirations interspersed with irregular apneic periods.

Ⓟ A patient remains conscious and aware during a simple partial seizure but will not be conscious or aware if they are having a complex partial seizure.

Ⓟ There is no cure for Amyotrophic Lateral Sclerosis, therefore treatment is purely symptomatic.

Ⓟ Treatment for viral meningitis is usually symptomatic, including antipyretics, analgesics and efforts to reduce intracranial pressure as needed.

Ⓟ Multiple sclerosis is an autoimmune disease where the body attacks and destroys the myelin sheath around the nerves resulting in decreased function of the affected nerves.

Ⓟ Inline spinal motion restriction is provided by placing the thumbs under the mandible and the index and middle fingers on the occipital ridges.

Ⓟ Ischemic strokes less than six hours old will have normal findings on computerized tomography, whereas hemorrhagic strokes will show hyperdensity around the area of the bleeding.

Ⓟ Multiple sclerosis is frequently a waxing and waning disorder that may be triggered by viruses, stress, and the spring and summer seasons.

Ⓟ The usual deterioration of respiratory patterns in increased intra-cranial pressure will follow an orderly pattern starting with bradyp-nea, then Cheyne-Stoke respirations, then central neurogenic hy-perventilation, then apneustic breathing.

Ⓟ Treatment options for a diffuse axonal injury include interventions to reduce intracranial pressure.

Ⓟ Spinal motion restriction involves in-line stabilization, application of a properly fitting cervical collar, placement of head blocks or equivalent, and body straps.

- Ⓟ Cluster headaches may be triggered by alcohol, histamine or nitro-glycerin.
- Ⓟ Tension headaches are often associated with depression, anxiety, premenstrual syndrome, fibromyalgia and other somatization disorders.
- Ⓟ Exacerbations of multiple sclerosis are marked by blurred or double vision, red-green distortion to the vision and blindness in one eye as well as weakness and difficulty with balance and coordination.
- Ⓟ Temporal lobe seizures start with an aura (foul smell, metallic or bitter taste or unusual hissing or ringing sounds) and odd visceral feelings in the chest/abdomen followed by automaticism.
- Ⓟ A subset of subarachnoid bleeds may not show up on computerized tomography and will require a lumbar puncture for definitive diagnosis.
- Ⓟ The initial onset of multiple sclerosis is generally between 20 and 40 years of age.

Ⓟ Nearly all brain injuries will cause hypertension. A brain injury with hypotension is a strong indicator that the patient has either another source of blood loss that need to be treated or is experiencing neurogenic shock.

Ⓟ Bradycardia, systolic hypertension and abnormal respirations are called Cushing's triad. This triad indicates severe intracranial pressure and often does not have a good outcome.

Ⓟ The three components of the Glasgow Coma Scale are motor response, verbal response and eye opening.

Ⓟ Patients with depressed and basilar skull fractures should receive antibiotics early in their course of treatment to reduce the risk of intracranial infection.

Ⓟ Movement and sensation of all extremities should be assessed before and after applying spinal stabilization.

Ⓟ Side effects of Rifampin (Rifadin) include red-orange urine and gastrointestinal upset. Although the drug is best taken on an empty stomach, it can be taken with food in cases of GI intolerance.

Ⓟ The occiput of a child under the age of eleven is prominent and may alter cervical spinal alignment when the child lies on a backboard. Padding should be placed under the shoulders.

Ⓟ Treatment for autonomic dysreflexia starts with treating the underlying cause. (Providing an enema for fecal impaction, relieving urinary catheter obstruction, etc.).

Ⓟ Rifampin (Rifadin) should not be given to pregnant women.

Ⓟ Function will usually resolve after an exacerbation of multiple sclerosis, but each remission will lead to some permanent dysfunction over time.

Ⓟ Cluster headaches are more common in the spring and fall.

- Ⓟ Airway is the primary concern for a seizing patient. Position them on their side and suction as needed. Apply oxygen as soon as possible.
- Ⓟ A Glasgow coma score of 13 – 15 is considered normal or mild brain injury, a score of 9 – 12 is moderate brain injury and a score of eight or less is considered profound brain injury.
- Ⓟ When placing padding under the shoulders of a pediatric patient who is immobilized on a backboard, the external auditory meatus should be in line with the shoulder.
- Ⓟ The backboard under a pregnant woman should be tipped 15 to 20 degrees to prevent venocaval compression syndrome.
- Ⓟ Patients with migraines or cluster headaches may find relief if cold packs are applied to the head, warm packs are preferred for tension headaches.
- Ⓟ Intravenous fluids should be administered judiciously to stroke patients to minimize intracranial pressure.

- Ⓟ There is no cure for multiple sclerosis. Steroids, beta-interferon and immunosuppressants may minimize symptoms of multiple sclerosis.
- Ⓟ Myasthenia Gravis is a disease which causes muscle weakness during activity with return of strength after rest.
- Ⓟ Two common causes of seizures include hypoglycemia and fever.
- Ⓟ To test the oculocephalic reflex, the patient's head is briskly rotated either left or right. If the eyes deviate away from the direction the head is rotated, it is considered a normal finding.
- Ⓟ Patients with spinal cord injuries in the cervical region may be unable to cough or clear secretions and may need frequent suctioning.
- Ⓟ High flow oxygen has been used to relieve the pain of a cluster headache.
- Ⓟ When assessing the oculocephalic reflex, if the eyes remain midline or move in a dysconjugate manner, this is an abnormal finding that indicates brainstem integrity is lost.

Ⓟ Never pack the ears or nose if there is a discharge containing cerebrospinal fluid to reduce the risk of increasing intracranial pressure.

Ⓟ Warn patients with increased ICP prior to touching them, use gentle movements, avoid jarring the bed, making loud noises or using bright lights to minimize spikes in intracranial pressure.

Ⓟ Spinal cord injuries may progress upwards due to edema. Respiratory status should be closely evaluated to assure that effort is not deteriorating and intubation is not required.

Ⓟ Hypertonic saline may be used to reduce intracranial pressure in stroke patients.

Ⓟ Antihypertensive therapy after a stroke is reserved for patients whose blood pressures climb above 185 systolic or 110 diastolic.

Ⓟ Rifampin (Rifadin) is known to inactivate birth control pills, therefore patients prescribed this medication should be encouraged to use alternate birth control methods.

Ⓟ The weakness of myasthenia gravis is almost always evident in the eye with symptoms such as drooping eyelid, double vision or difficulty keeping the eye closed.

Ⓟ Benzodiazepines, specifically Diazepam (Valium) or Lorazepam (Ativan) intravenously or rectally, are usually chosen to stop seizure activity.

Ⓟ Once seizure activity has stopped, anticonvulsants such as Phenytoin (Dilantin), Phenobarbital and Fosphenytoin Sodium (Cerebyx) are considered to prevent recurrence.

Ⓟ The weakness of myasthenia gravis may cause difficulty with swallowing or speech.

Ⓟ In severe cases of myasthenia gravis, a patient may experience respiratory paralysis and arrest.

Ⓟ Labetalol (Normodyne, Trandate) is frequently chosen to reduce blood pressure after a stroke.

Ⓟ rt-PA (Alteplase) is the only fibrinolytic drug which has been approved by the Federal Drug Administration (FDA) for the treatment of ischemic strokes.

Ⓟ Administration of edrophonium (Tensilon) will temporarily improve the symptoms of myasthenia gravis.

Ⓟ The doll's eye test should not be performed on patients with suspected cervical spinal injuries.

Ⓟ The oculovestibular reflex is also known as the water caloric test.

Ⓟ Pain may increase intracranial pressure, therefore prophylactically administer pain medications to brain injured patients.

Ⓟ Amyotrophic Lateral Sclerosis does not affect cognitive function or the ability to move the eyes.

Ⓟ The doll's eye test is used to test the oculocephalic reflex.

- Ⓟ The symptoms of Parkinson's disease may be remembered with the mnemonic TRAP. (T – tremor, R – rigidity of muscles, A – akinesia and bradykinesia, and P - postural instability).
- Ⓟ Other symptoms of Parkinson's disease include depression, difficulty swallowing or speaking, urinary problems or constipation, and sleep disruptions.
- Ⓟ Myasthenia gravis is controlled with pyridostigmine bromide (Mestinon), barbiturates, opiates, quinidine, quinine, corticotrophin, corticosteroids, aminoglycosides, and muscle relaxants.
- Ⓟ Treatment of status epilepticus involves intubation and mechanical ventilation as well as large doses of benzodiazepines and anticonvulsants to stop and control seizure activity.
- Ⓟ Parkinson's disease usually starts after the age of 50 and is progressive with cumulative loss of function.
- Ⓟ Fibrinolytic therapy is indicated for ischemic strokes but contraindicated for hemorrhagic strokes.

ⓟ Never insert anything, including nasogastric tubes and nasopharyngeal trumpets, in the nares of a patient suspected of having a basilar skull fracture.

ⓟ To perform the water caloric test, ice water is injected into the ear of the unresponsive patient. If both eyes move towards the ear into which the water was instilled, it is considered a normal finding.

ⓟ The action of suctioning may actually increase intracranial pressure, therefore administration of intravenous or endotracheal lidocaine (xylocaine) prior to suctioning may decrease this effect.

ⓟ Early in the disease process, the tremor of Parkinson's disease is usually unilateral and increases with rest. It becomes less noticeable with movement.

ⓟ Patients with basilar skull fractures should be discouraged from sneezing or coughing and nasal cannulas should be avoided to prevent a pneumocephalus.

- ⓟ Frequent interventions for patients with spinal cord injuries include urinary catheters, gastric tubes and histamine-two blockers.
- ⓟ Ideally, fibrinolytic therapy is initiated within three hours of onset of stroke symptoms.
- ⓟ The dose of rt-PA (Alteplase) after an ischemic stroke is 0.9 mg/kg, up to a maximum of 90 mg.
- ⓟ Treatment for subarachnoid bleeding includes aggressive efforts to reduce intracranial pressure. Calcium channel blockers may also be used to reduce cerebral blood vessel spasms and improve circulation.
- ⓟ The three meninges around the brain are the dura (outermost), the arachnoid (the middle layer) and the pia (the innermost).
- ⓟ Ganglionic blockers such as Hydralazine (Apresoline) are used to lower the blood pressure of patients in autonomic dysreflexia.
- ⓟ Drugs used to treat Parkinson's disease either stimulate dopamine production in the brain or replace dopamine in the brain.

- Ⓟ Women with migraine headaches should be taught to avoid oral contraceptives.
- Ⓟ When performing the water caloric test, if both eyes do not move towards the ice water, there is likely an interruption in the functional connection between the medulla and the mid-brain.
- Ⓟ Therapies (aside from pharmacological agents) used for headaches may include biofeedback, relaxation training, assertiveness training, family and dietary counseling and allergy testing.
- Ⓟ When intubating the patient with Gullian Barré syndrome, succinylcholine should not be administered to prevent lethal hyperkalemia.
- Ⓟ Pharmacological agents used to treat a tension headache include NSAIDs, narcotic analgesics, tricyclic antidepressants and selective serotonin uptake inhibitors.
- Ⓟ General anesthetic may be required as a last resort to stop muscular activities in cases of status epilepticus.

ⓟ Patients in neurogenic shock lose body heat and are prone to hypothermia, therefore, they should be covered and their body temperature closely monitored.

ⓟ The water caloric test should not be performed on patients with
tympanic membrane rupture. The test should also be avoided in
semi-conscious or conscious patients as it can stimulate dizziness
and vomiting.

ⓟ The head of the bed should be elevated for patients with autonomic dysreflexia to reduce intracranial pressure.

ⓟ Patients with subarachnoid bleeds require surgical repair of the deficit as well as evacuation of the blood from the subarachnoid
space.

ⓟ Angiography with stent placement is an alternative to fibrinolytic
therapy considered for ischemic strokes.

ⓟ Cervical spinal stabilization should be implemented simultaneously
with airway assessments in cases of trauma.

- ⓟ 10% of the dose of rt-PA (Alteplase) is given immediately as a bolus, followed by 90% of the drug as an intravenous infusion over one hour.
- ⓟ Infants and children with increased intracranial pressure may exhibit vomiting, anorexia, poor feeding, high-pitched cries and bulging fontanelles.
- ⓟ Infants and children with increased intracranial pressure may develop "sun setting eyes", where the pupils deviate downwards causing the sclera to become prominent in the upper parts of the eye.
- ⓟ Biot's respirations are rapid deep respirations punctuated with long periods of apnea sometimes associated with increased intracranial pressure.
- ⓟ The symptoms of a cerebral contusion may be delayed by hours or days and may include personality changes, nausea, vomiting, deficits in behavior and motor function, language deficits and visual disturbances.

Ⓟ To assess posterior cord function, use a cotton wisp (to assess light touch) or a turning fork (to assess vibration).

Ⓟ To assess for proprioception deficits, have a patient close his or her eyes and move the great toe into various positions. Ask the patient to identify the position the toe has been moved.

Ⓟ Proprioception is affected by injuries to the posterior cord.

Ⓟ Second impact syndrome occurs when an individual sustains a second concussion before the effects of the first concussion have healed. This syndrome can be fatal.

Ⓟ To reduce the incidence of second impact syndrome, encourage individuals who have sustained a concussion to avoid high risk activities until cleared by a provider.

Ⓟ When assessing for sensory deficits after a spinal cord injury, always start from areas of decreased sensation and move towards areas of increased sensation (patients are more sensitive to the appearance of sensation than the disappearance of sensation.)

Ⓟ To assess for deficits associated with lateral cord injuries, use the broken end of a wooden cotton tipped applicator (to assess for pain).

Ⓟ Factors which depress the sympathetic center of the brain such as brain injuries, brain hypoxia, overdose of CNS depressants, and hypoglycemia can cause neurogenic shock.

Ⓟ Clinical indications of neurogenic shock may include priapism, decreased core body temperature, bradycardia, and bradypnea.

Ⓟ Patients with spinal cord injuries who develop neurogenic shock may be cool and clammy above the level of the injury with warm dry skin below the level of the injury.

Ⓟ Signs of neurogenic shock are the opposite of hypovolemic shock.

Ⓟ Neurogenic shock is treated with fluid boluses to restore blood pressure. If fluid boluses are ineffective, vasopressors may be added.

- Ⓟ A common vasopressor used in the treatment of neurogenic shock is neosynephrine (Phenylephrine), an alpha-adrenergic receptor stimulant.
- Ⓟ Patients with bradycardia secondary to neurogenic shock are treated with atropine.
- Ⓟ The bradypnea and inadequate respiratory effort associated with neurogenic shock is usually treated with intubation and mechanical ventilation.
- Ⓟ Headaches which increase in intensity over a period of time may be indicative of a space occupying lesion, such as a tumor.
- Ⓟ If an entire family develops headaches, consider the possibility of carbon monoxide poisoning.
- Ⓟ Headaches in patients on treatment for cancer, those with immunosuppressive illnesses or on immunosuppressive drugs should raise the index of suspicion for meningitis.

- ℗ Dilantin should be missed with normal saline rather than a dextrose containing solution when administering intravenously.
- ℗ Dilantin is very alkali. Infiltration can cause severe tissue necrosis.
- ℗ If Dilantin is given to rapidly, it may cause hypotension, heart blocks and bradycardia. Never give Dilantin faster than 50 mg/minute (do not exceed 25 mg/minute in the elderly).
- ℗ Side effects of Phenobarbital include respiratory suppression, CNS depression and hypotension.
- ℗ When administering Fosphenytion Sodium (Cerebyx), watch the cardiac monitor, blood pressure and respirations during the infusion and up to 20 minutes after the infusion.
- ℗ Fosphenytion Sodium (Cerebyx) can be given via the intramuscular route if intravenous access is not available.
- ℗ The symptoms of multiple sclerosis may be controlled by steroids, beta-interferon and immunosupressants.

- Ⓟ Fosphenytion Sodium (Cerebyx) can be given via the intramuscular route if intravenous access is not available.
- Ⓟ The symptoms of myasthenia gravis often begin between the ages of 20 and 30 years.
- Ⓟ Females develop myasthenia gravis more than male. There is a familial tendency to the disease.
- Ⓟ Aside from fatigue, the symptoms of myasthenia gravis are more common in hot weather, with infection, or with ingestion of psychotropic drugs, antibiotics and anti-dysrhythmic drugs.

Bibliography for neurological emergencies

Andreoni, C. (2013). Pediatric Considerations in Emergency Nursing. In B. B. Hammond, & P. Gerber-Zimmerman (Eds.), *Sheehy's Emergency Nursing: Principals and Practice* (7 ed., pp. 547 - 570). Philadelphia: Elsevier.

Bhatia, K., & Sharma, R. (2013). Eye Emergencies. In J. G. Adams, *Emergency Medicine* (pp. 209 - 225). Philadelphia: Elsevier.

Everson, F.P. (2013). Spinal Cord and Neck Trauma. In B. B. Hammond, & P. Gerber-Zimmerman (Eds.), *Sheehy's Emergency Nursing: Principals and Practice* (7 ed., pp. 395 - 406). Philadelphia: Elsevier.

Heegaard, W. G. and Biros M.H. (2014). Head Injury. In J. A. Marx, R. S. Hockberger, & R. M. Walls, *Rosen's Emergency Medicine* (pp. 339 - 367). Philadelphia: Elsevier

McLaughlin, J.C. (2013). Head Injuries. In B. B. Hammond, & P. Gerber-Zimmerman (Eds.), *Sheehy's Emergency Nursing: Principals and Practice* (7 ed., pp. 379 - 393). Philadelphia: Elsevier.

McMullan, J. T., Duvivier, E. H., Pollack, C.V. (2014). Seizure Disorders. In J. A. Marx, R. S. Hockberger, & R. M. Walls, *Rosen's Emergency Medicine* (8 ed., pp1375 - 1385). Philadelphia: Elsevier.

National Institute of Health. (no date). *Multiple Sclerosis*. Retrieved January 21, 2016, from PubMed Health: http://www.ncbi.nlm.nih.gov/pubmedhealth/PMHT0024311/

National Institute of Neurological Disorders and Stroke. (2015, July 27). *Myasthenia Gravis Fact Sheet*. Retrieved January 21, 2016, from National Institute of Neurological Disorders and Stroke: http://www.ninds.nih.gov/disorders/myasthenia_gravis/detail_myasthenia_gravis.htm

Perez-Barcena, J., Llompart-Pou, J. A., & O'Phelan, K. H. (2014, October 10). Intracranial Pressure Monitoring and Management of Intracranial Hypertension. *Critical Care Clinics, 30* (4), 730 - 750.

Pioro, E. P., Saver, D. F., Scherger, J. E., Ferri, F. F., Misulis, K. E., Satya-Murti, S., & McNeil, D. E. (2011, June 22). *Amyotrophic lateral sclerosis*. Retrieved 21 January, from First Consult: https://www.clinicalkey.com/#!/content/medical_topic/21-s2.0-1014439

Shepherd Center and KPK Interactive. (2011). *Understanding Spinal Cord Injury.* Atlanta: Shepherd Center.

Singh, A., Promes, S. B. (2013). Meningitis, Enxcephalitis, and Brain Abscess. In J. G. Adams, *Emergency Medicine* (2 ed., pp. 1443 - 1453). Philadelphia: Elsevier.

Walsh, R. (2013) Neurological Emergencies. In B. B. Hammond, & P. Gerber-Zimmerman (Eds.), *Sheehy's Emergency Nursing: Principals and Practice* (7 ed., pp. 265 - 274). Philadelphia: Elsevier.

Ocular Emergencies

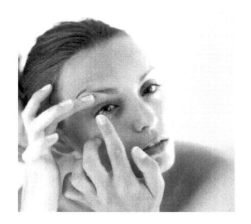

- ℗ Visual acuity should be done with contact lenses or glasses in place whenever possible.
- ℗ A cycloplegic is a medication which dilates and paralyzes the pupil.
- ℗ A thrombus or embolism in the central retinal artery or a branch of that artery is referred to as a central retinal artery occlusion.
- ℗ A collection of blood in the anterior chamber of the eye is termed a hyphema.
- ℗ When the neurosensory layers of the retina detach from the underlying choroid layer, it is called a retinal detachment.
- ℗ An injury to the outer layer of the cornea by foreign objects, contact lenses or exposure to ultraviolet light is termed a corneal abrasion.
- ℗ The globe may rupture due to mechanisms of injury which increase intraocular pressure or secondary to penetrating objects such as a pencil or dart.

Ⓟ Ocular burns caused by acids tend to be non-progressive and superficial because acids cause protein coagulation and limit further penetration into the structures of the eye.

Ⓟ Alkaline substances splashed in the eye rapidly combine with cellular lipids and produce coagulation necrosis with total cellular disruption.

Ⓟ Alkali substances can burn through the anterior chamber and injure underlying structures such as the iris and ciliary body in a very short period of time.

Ⓟ To remove contact lenses from dry eyes, instill saline drops and wait a few minutes before lens removal to prevent corneal damage.

Ⓟ Visual acuity should be performed as part of the initial assessment for all ocular complaints. The only exception is chemical burns to the eye. Flushing of the eye should precede measurement of visual acuity.

- Ⓟ Obtain a baseline pH using litmus paper prior to initiating irrigation of a chemically burned eye.
- Ⓟ Glaucoma is a buildup of aqueous fluid in the anterior chamber of the eye.
- Ⓟ Conjunctivitis is an infection of the conjunctiva.
- Ⓟ Keratitis is an infection of the cornea.
- Ⓟ Iritis is an infection of the iris and ciliary body, the part of the eye that slides over the lens to create the size and shape of the pupil.
- Ⓟ Untreated glaucoma may lead to permanent visual impairment or vision loss.
- Ⓟ Risk factors for a central retinal artery occlusion includes a history of valvular heart disease or atrial fibrillation.
- Ⓟ Conjunctivitis may be caused by bacterial or viral infections, chlamydia, allergic reactions, chemical burns, foreign bodies in the eye, and exposure to irritants.

- Ⓟ An erosion of the outer layer of the cornea is known as a corneal ulceration.
- Ⓟ The pupil of a ruptured globe may assume a tear drop or pointed shape with the point directed towards the site of the rupture.
- Ⓟ Examples of alkali substances that may be splashed into the eye include lye, cement, lime, and ammonia; as well as the residue from sparklers and flares.
- Ⓟ If a contact lens needs to be removed due to injury or burn and it won't easily come off, slide it off the cornea to the sclera and maintain it in that position until removed by a physician.
- Ⓟ A frequent cause of keratitis is ultraviolet burns.
- Ⓟ Keratitis caused by ultraviolent light often begins six to ten hours after exposure to sources such as welding arcs, sun tanning beds, reading on the beach, ice climbing or snow skiing without appropriate eye protection.
- Ⓟ Hyphemas may be spontaneous or may follow trauma to the eye.

- ℗ Iritis is caused by infections such as rheumatic diseases, ankylosing spondylitis, or syphilis. Iritis may also follow traumatic eye injuries.
- ℗ When testing visual acuity, each eye should be tested separately first, then together, testing the unaffected eye first to serve as a control.
- ℗ Symptoms of glaucoma include severe sudden-onset deep unilateral eye pain that may be accompanied by a headache, abdominal pain, nausea and vomiting.
- ℗ During acute glaucoma, a patient may describe seeing a halo around lights. Visual acuity will usually be diminished.
- ℗ The onset of symptoms of glaucoma often occurs when a patient is in a darkened environment such as watching television in the dark or reading in poor lighting.
- ℗ Manifestations of conjunctivitis include purulent or mucopurulent discharge with matting of the eyelids in the morning and a gritty sensation in the affected eye.

- Ⓟ Keratitis frequently causes photophobia and corneal irregularity as well as severe eye pain.
- Ⓟ Conjunctivitis can spread from one person to another easily through contact.
- Ⓟ Causes of retinal detachment include trauma, aging, hypertension, and diabetes.
- Ⓟ A corneal abrasion which is invaded by bacteria may become a corneal ulceration. Corneal ulcerations may also develop when the cornea is allowed to dry out (e.g. Bell's Palsy).
- Ⓟ The pupil of a patient with iritis is usually small, irregular and sluggish to react. The cornea may appear hazy.
- Ⓟ Never instill medications into the eye of patient wearing contact lenses as the medication can combine chemically with the contact and cause eye irritation or lens damage.
- Ⓟ All chemical splashes to the eye should be immediately irrigated, do not delay irrigation for any reason.

- Ⓟ Patients with ruptured globes will have varying degrees of visual disturbances, depending on the extent of the injury. These disturbances range from blurry vision to complete blindness.
- Ⓟ Central retinal artery occlusions can lead to permanent blindness if the blood clot causing the condition is not relieved within one to two hours, therefore this condition must be treated with urgency.
- Ⓟ Recent exposure to ultraviolet light (welding arcs, sun lamps, or glare off of ice or snow), and foreign bodies in the eye can lead to corneal abrasions and ultimately ulcerations.
- Ⓟ Symptoms of keratitis include blurred vision, intense photophobia, lacrimation, and pain when pressure is applied to the eye.
- Ⓟ To flush the eye, the upper eyelid is everted, and copious amounts of normal saline or lactated Ringers's solution should be run into the eye.
- Ⓟ The eye of a patient with keratitis is usually patched for 24 hours to allow the cornea to heal. Cycloplegics may be instilled in the eye.

- ℗ Because iritis is an infection deep in the eye, it is treated with non-steroidal anti-inflammatory drugs. Cycloplegics may also be administered.
- ℗ The eye that has been burned by a chemical should be flushed until the pH of the surface of the eye is neutral (pH approximately 7.4—7.6) as determined by litmus paper.
- ℗ Globe ruptures may cause the anterior chamber to bulge or it may cause it to be flat, depending on the location of the rupture.
- ℗ Symptoms of a corneal abrasion or ulceration include pain in the eye with redness, blinking and tearing. The patient may verbalize a foreign body-type sensation.
- ℗ Patients with hyphemas should be discouraged from performing activities such as bending forward, blowing the nose, sneezing or performing Valsalva's maneuver.
- ℗ After flushing an eye burned by chemicals; topical antibiotics, cycloplegic agents, and steroids may be prescribed.

Ⓟ The Snellen eye chart is used to test vision on patients who can recognize letters in the English language.

Ⓟ Acuity may be tested on a "E" chart or a picture chart if the patient is not familiar with letters of the English language and for young children.

Ⓟ Regardless of the type of eye chart used, the patient should stand twenty feet from the chart to ensure accuracy.

Ⓟ Patients with iritis may find relief from the application of warm compresses to the affected eye.

Ⓟ The eye affected by glaucoma may appear reddened and the pupil on the affected side may be mid-position, poorly reactive, or even fixed.

Ⓟ Conjunctivitis is treated with antibiotic ointment or antibiotic drops.

Ⓟ Patients with a hyphema may complain of pain to the front of the eye and a reddish hue to their vision. Blood may be visualized in the anterior chamber of the eye.

Ⓟ Retinal detachments require prompt medical attention to prevent permanent vision loss.

Ⓟ Secure any object protruding from a ruptured globe by either covering it (e.g. a paper cup) or securing it (e.g. gauze rolls).

Ⓟ Mydriatic, cycloplegic, and steroid drops should be used in caution with the elderly because they may induce angle-closure glaucoma.

Ⓟ Patients with a retinal detachment will frequently describe a curtain or veil that partially obscures the upper part of the visual field.

Ⓟ Drugs used in the treatment of a central retinal artery occlusion include anticoagulants, thrombolytics, acetazolamide (Diamox), and low molecular-weight dextran.

Ⓟ Never place pressure or tight dressings over an eye that may have a foreign object in it.

Ⓟ When flushing an eye, direct the flow of the irrigant onto the conjunctiva from the inner to outer canthus avoiding directing the stream at the cornea.

- ℗ During eye irrigation, the patient should roll their eyes in all directions during flushing to ensure the entire eye is irrigated.
- ℗ To reduce the risk of cross-contamination, patients with conjunctivitis should be instructed to avoid using eye make-up or contacts during the infection.
- ℗ A Rosenbaum eye chart can be used when a patient cannot stand 20 feet from another form of eye chart. The Rosenbaum eye chart is held 14 inches from the patient's face.
- ℗ Normal intraocular pressure is less than 20 mmHg. During glaucoma, intraocular pressures may elevate as high as 40 to 80 mmHg.
- ℗ When securing an object imbedded in a globe, patch the unaffected eye to decrease the risk of injury secondary to consensual movement.
- ℗ Never place eye drops or ointments into an eye which may be ruptured, as they could be absorbed through the rupture site.

Ⓟ Discharge teaching for a patient with conjunctivitis should include removal of crusting on the eyelids by applying baby shampoo, starting from the inside of the eyelid and moving outwards.

Ⓟ Patients with iritis need to be encouraged to stay in darkened environments and wear sunglasses when exposed to light to decrease the discomfort of photophobia.

Ⓟ Carbogen gas is sometimes used in the treatment of a central retinal artery occlusion.

Ⓟ Carbogen gas is a canister of gas containing 95% oxygen plus 5% carbon dioxide that causes vasodilation. It must be used with caution in patients with chronic obstructive pulmonary disease.

Ⓟ Pilocarpine eye drops (such as Pilocar or Pilogel) or beta-adrenergic eye drops may be administered to decrease intraocular pressure in a patient with glaucoma.

Ⓟ When a retina detaches, the patient may experience a brilliant flash of lights in the visual field followed by visualization of floaters.

- Ⓟ If visual charts are inaccessible, stand 20 feet from the patient, hold up fingers and ask the patient to count the fingers. If they cannot count, step one foot closer and record the distance at which the patient can accurately count the number of fingers.
- Ⓟ Patients with hyphemas should be cared for with the head of the bed elevated.
- Ⓟ Pharmacological agents for corneal abrasions and ulcerations include topical ophthalmic anesthesia, cycloplegic drops, and ophthalmic antibiotics.
- Ⓟ Maintain the patient with a ruptured globe in the Semi-Fowler's position to reduce intraocular pressure.
- Ⓟ After flushing an eye following a chemical splash, check the pH of the eye both at the conclusion of flushing and again 20 minutes later, as chemical residue from the deep inside the eye may surface and additional flushing may be required.

Ⓟ Eye drops should be administered in the conjunctival sac at the center of the lower lid rather than directly onto the cornea.

Ⓟ If a patient is unable to see an eye chart, record the distance at which a patient can detect hand motion. If a patient cannot see hand motion, record if light perception exists or not.

Ⓟ Teach patients with iritis to apply warm compresses to the eye to control pain.

Ⓟ Osmotic diuretics such as mannitol (Osmitrol) may be used to decrease body fluid in a patient with glaucoma thereby decreasing intraocular pressure.

Ⓟ Analgesics are given to reduce the pain of a hyphema. NSAIDs and aspirin are avoided to reduce the risk of renewed or continued bleeding associated with the condition.

Ⓟ While patients await repair of a retinal detachment by an ophthalmologist, maintain bed rest. Both eyes should be bilaterally patched to decrease eye movement.

℗ Encourage patients with corneal ulcerations and abrasions to wear sunglasses and stay in darkened environments to reduce photophobia.

℗ Instill topical ophthalmic anesthetic into the affected eye prior to flushing an eye unless a globe rupture is suspected. Do not instill more than one drop at a time, which can increase tearing and decrease the concentration of the medication.

Bibliography for ocular emergencies

Amsterdam, J. T. (2014). Oral Medicine. In J. A. Marx, R. S. Hockberger, & R. M. Walls, *Rosen's Emergency Medicine* (pp. 895 - 908). Philadelphia: Elsevier.

Andreoni, C. (2013). Pediatric Considerations in Emergency Nursing. In B. B. Hammond, & P. Gerber-Zimmerman (Eds.), *Sheehy's Emergency Nursing: Principals and Practice* (7 ed., pp. 547 - 570). Philadelphia: Elsevier.

Asensio, J. A., & Trunkey, D. D. (2016). Initial Assessment and Resuscitation. In *Therapy of Trauma and Surgical Critical Care* (2 ed., pp. 57 - 69). Philadelphia: Elsevier.

Bhatia, K., & Sharma, R. (2013). Eye Emergencies. In J. G. Adams, *Emergency Medicine* (pp. 209 - 225). Philadelphia: Elsevier.

Centers for Disease Control and Prevention. (2014, January 9). *Conjunctivitis (Pink Eye)*. Retrieved from Centers for Disease Control and Prevention: http://www.cdc.gov/conjunctivitis/clinical.html

Chi, J. J., & Alam, D. S. (2014). Facial Trauma. In J. L. Cameron, & A. M. Cameron, *Current Surgical Therapy* (11 ed., pp. 1070 - 1081). Philadelphia: Elsevier.

Dahl, A. A. (2015, May 14). *Keratitis*. Retrieved from MedicineNet.com: http://www.medicinenet.com/keratitis/article.htm

Egging, D. (2013). Facial, ENT, and Dental Emergencies. In B. B. Hammond, & P. Gerber-Zimmerman (Eds.), *Sheehy's Emergency Nursing: Principals and Practice* (7 ed., pp. 275 - 289). Philadelphia: Elsevier.

Mays, M., Kabongo, M. L., & Satya-Murti, S. (January 31, 2012). *Trigeminal Neuralgia*. Retrieved from First Consult: https://www.clinicalkey.com/#!/content/medical_topic/21-s2.0-1014499

Misulis, K. E., Galloway, G. M., & Harper, W. (2010, August 10). *Bell's Palsy*. Retrieved from First Consult: https://www.clinicalkey.com/#!/content/medical_topic/21-s2.0-1014441

Muchatuta, M. N. (2015, December 14). *Iritis and Uveitis*. Retrieved from MedScape: http://emedicine.medscape.com/article/798323-overview

National Institutes of Health. (2010, July). *Meniere's Disease*. Retrieved from National Institute on Deafness and Other Communication Disorders: http://www.nidcd.nih.gov/health/balance/pages/meniere.aspx

Peng, L. F. (2014, December 31). *Avulsed Tooth Treatment and Management*. Retrieved from MedScape: http://emedicine.medscape.com/article/763291-treatment

Watkins, T. A., Opie , N. J., & Norman, A. (2011, August 1). Airway choices in maxillofacial trauma. *Trends in Anesthesia and Critical Care, 1*(4), 179 – 190

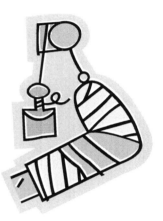

Orthopedic Emergencies

- Ⓟ Ice should be applied to contusions and hematomas for the first 48 hours, than heat is applied to aid absorption of the blood.
- Ⓟ Multiple contusions or hematomas from minor mechanisms of injury may indicate a hematological disorder. A coagulation panel should be drawn.
- Ⓟ A sprain is an injury to a ligament, a strain is an injury to a muscle or tendon.
- Ⓟ Crutches should always be fitted with the patient wearing a shoe on the unaffected foot to assure proper sizing.
- Ⓟ Costochondritis is an acute, self-limiting inflammation of the costal cartilage where the ribs and sternum come together.
- Ⓟ Bursitis may be caused by repetitive use of a joint or invasion of bacteria and fungus in the bursal sac.
- Ⓟ Arthritis is a chronic degeneration of the cartilage over the ends of bones.
- Ⓟ A collection of fluid in the joint space is known as a joint effusion.

Ⓟ The knee is the most common joint where effusions develop.

Ⓟ Subluxation of a joint is defined as joint ends being out of alignment, but the bone ends are still in contact.

Ⓟ Dislocation of a joint is defined as an injury where not only the bone ends are out of alignment, but they are no longer in contact.

Ⓟ The usual mechanism of injury of an anterior shoulder dislocation is falling on outstretched hands.

Ⓟ The ulnar nerve innervates the pinky finger, the inside of the ring finger and the side of the palm opposite the thumb.

Ⓟ Damage to the ulnar nerve diminishes the ability of the patient to fan their fingers. The pinky and ring finger will be limp.

Ⓟ The median nerve innervates most of the palm of the hand, the middle and index finger and part of the ring finger.

Ⓟ Damage to the median nerve diminishes the patient's ability to bring their thumb across the palm of the hand to the pinky finger.

- Ⓟ The radial nerve innervates the base of the thumb on both the front and back of the hand.
- Ⓟ Damage to the radial nerve alters the ability of the patient to hold their thumb up in the hitch-hikers sign.
- Ⓟ An open fracture is one in which the bone is either protruding from the skin or the bone protruded at the time of the injury but retracted afterwards.
- Ⓟ Drivers are the most likely to be injured in a motor vehicle collision.
- Ⓟ Passengers travelling in the backseat of a vehicle are least likely to be seriously injured.
- Ⓟ Fractures of the knee often involve the peroneal or tibial nerve and the popliteal artery.
- Ⓟ Non-displaced patellar fractures are usually placed in a long leg cylinder cast; displaced fractures usually require surgery.
- Ⓟ Closed pelvic fractures carry a mortality of 8 to 10%, open pelvic fractures carry a mortality of 40 to 60%.

Ⓟ Increased pressures within a muscle compartment cause compartment syndrome.

Ⓟ Signs of osteomyelitis include erythema, warmth, swelling and pain to the area of infection.

Ⓟ Tractions splints are applied to diminish pain and control bleeding.

Ⓟ Intrusion into a passenger compartment is a strong predictor of injury. The greater the intrusion into the passenger compartment, the higher the risk of injury.

Ⓟ Tourniquets should be promptly applied to amputations or injuries with significant blood loss.

Ⓟ Ankles, knees and shoulders are the most susceptible to sprains.

Ⓟ Costochondritis usually occurs with physical exertion or repetitive movements and may affect one rib junction or multiple rib junctions.

- ⓅBursitis causes pain, redness, and swelling with limited range of motion over the affected bursa. It will also be warm to touch.
- ⓅMen often develop arthritis before the age of 45, women after 55.
- ⓅHemophilia can result in a collection of blood in a joint space.
- ⓅPosterior shoulder dislocations are rare and may occur with seizures or a strong blow to the front of the shoulder.
- ⓅPatellar dislocation results in a flexed knee with the patella palpated lateral to the femoral condyle.
- ⓅThe peroneal nerve innervates the top of the foot. Damage to this nerve causes loss of sensation to the top of the foot and inability to raise the foot up.
- ⓅThe tibial nerve innervates the bottom of the foot. Damage to this nerve causes loss of sensation to the bottom of the foot and inability to push the foot down.

- ℗ Foreign objects which penetrate the skin causing fractures are classified as open fractures.
- ℗ Avulsion fractures are usually associated with severe strains in which the overstretched tendon pulls a bone chip off its insertion point.
- ℗ A torus fracture is a compression fracture where the fractured bone ends are pushed into one another but the cortical margins on the outside of the bone are untouched.
- ℗ Radial and ulnar fractures at the wrist which angulate upwards are known as Colle's fractures and appear in the shape of a fork when the arm is viewed from the side.
- ℗ Radial and ulnar fractures at the wrist which angulate downward are known as Smith's fractures and appear in the shape of a hoe when the arm is viewed from the side.
- ℗ Ice should not be applied to limbs affected by compartment syndrome.

Ⓟ Ejection from a vehicle significantly increases the odds of death or serious injury.

Ⓟ Patients with osteomyelitis complain of pain when the affected bone is palpated and will have decreased range of motion in areas dependent on that bone.

Ⓟ Ⓟ External compression of a muscle compartment from circumferential casts, splint or tape, elastic bandages, or military anti-shock trousers (MAST pants) can cause compartment syndrome.

Ⓟ The top of properly fitted crutches should be 1 to 1 ½ inches below the axilla when the crutches are at a 25 degree angle with the body (6 to 8 inches on either side of the feet).

Ⓟ First degree (mild) sprains and strains should have a compression bandage applied, be intermittently elevated with cold packs for 12 hours and the patient instructed to undertake light weight-bearing only.

- (P) If an occupant in a vehicle is either injured or killed, there is an increased risk that other occupants will have significant injury.
- (P) Second degree (moderate) sprains and strains should have a compression bandage applied, be intermittently elevated with cold packs for 24 hours and the patient instructed to undertake light weight bearing only.
- (P) Third degree (severe) sprains and strains will require splinting or casting with elevation for 24 – 72 hours and no weight-bearing. Surgery is required for complete ruptures or tears.
- (P) The pain related to bursitis of the shoulder may radiate up the neck and down to the fingertips.
- (P) Repetitive use of a tendon can cause an inflammation of the tendon known as tendinitis.
- (P) The pain of arthritis is usually worse as the day progresses.
- (P) Substance abuse increases the risk of septic arthritis with joint effusions.

Ⓟ Before treatment, an anterior shoulder dislocation will cause abduction and the patient will be unable to bring the elbow down to
the chest or touch the opposite ear with the hand.

Ⓟ On arrival, a patient with a posterior shoulder dislocation will hold
their arm to their side and be unable to rotate it externally.

Ⓟ It is essential to compare pulses in the injured extremity with pulses
in the unaffected extremity to assure that decreased pulse quality
is not due to underlying disease rather than acute injury.

Ⓟ Speed is a strong contributor to injury. The faster a vehicle is moving at the time of a collision, the greater the likelihood that occupants of that vehicle will be injured.

Ⓟ Any open area over a fracture site should be treated as a compound
fracture.

Ⓟ When one surface of a bone is broken but the other surface is in-
tact, it is called a greenstick fracture. This is most common in children.

Ⓟ A frequent mechanism of injury for scaphoid fractures is falling on the outstretched hand.

Ⓟ Traction splints are suitable for mid-shaft femur fractures or fractures of the upper third of the tibia, but not for hip, lower tibia, lower fibula, or ankle fractures.

Ⓟ Traction splints should not be applied to a femur fracture with concomitant tibia/fibula fractures.

Ⓟ Bleeding into muscle compartments from injury, fractures, vascular trauma or blood dyscrasias such as hemophilia are common causes of compartment syndrome.

Ⓟ Overuse of a muscle compartment from forced marches or long distance running can cause intercompartmental edema leading to compartment syndrome.

Ⓟ If osteomyelitis is suspected, the infected area should be immobilized, intravenous antibiotics initiated as prescribed, and isolation precautions initiated.

- Ⓟ Leaning on the elbow for significant periods of time may cause bursitis of the elbow.
- Ⓟ Arthritis causes stiffness of the affected joint with inactivity and increased pain on repetitive movement.
- Ⓟ A fall from three times a victim's height or greater should raise the concern for significant injury.
- Ⓟ The inflammation of gout can contribute to a joint effusion.
- Ⓟ Joint injuries frequently have associated neurovascular involvement and must be reduced as soon as possible to prevent permanent damage.
- Ⓟ A sling and swath bandage or shoulder immobilizer is applied after reduction of anterior and posterior shoulder dislocations.
- Ⓟ Partially amputated limbs should be splinted in anatomical position.
- Ⓟ Care of an open fracture includes wound cleansing with normal saline irrigation followed by application of a dry sterile dressing.

Ⓟ Compartment syndrome may be caused by edema within a muscle compartment from venomous snake or spider bites, electrical burns, hypothermia or frostbite.

Ⓟ Bacteriostatic solutions should not be applied to open fractures because if they come into contact with the bone ends, it may delay bone healing.

Ⓟ Wound cultures should be obtained prior to cleansing an open fracture.

Ⓟ Because of the high risk of osteomyelitis, prophylactic antibiotics will almost always be prescribed for open fractures.

Ⓟ Fractures may have significant associated blood loss; always assess for hypovolemia.

Ⓟ Because of the strength of the femur bone, femur fractures usually involve trauma to other bones or body systems.

- Ⓟ Patients with clavicular fractures will not raise the affected arm and tend to tilt their head towards the side of the injury with the chin directed in the opposite direction.
- Ⓟ Scaphoid fractures usually have wrist pain and increased pain when pressure is applied to the indentation at the base of the thumb (sometimes referred to as the "snuff box").
- Ⓟ Circumferential burns in skin around a muscle compartment or hematomas around a muscle compartment may cause compartment syndrome.
- Ⓟ Rhabdomyolysis is caused by the release of myoglobin from injured muscles into the circulation.
- Ⓟ Injection of substances under pressure, such as from a paint or grease gun, can lead to compartment syndrome in the muscle compartment into which the substance is injected.
- Ⓟ Assess areas around and distal to hematomas and contusions for neurovascular compromise and compartment syndrome.

Ⓟ Cold packs should be applied to injured areas for 20 minutes at a time during the first 48 hours to promote vasoconstriction and reduce swelling.

Ⓟ 48 hours after an injury, patients need to be instructed to switch from cold packs to heat to encourage vasodilation and re-absorption of edema.

Ⓟ The hand pieces of the crutches should be fitted so that the elbow is at a 30 degree angle of flexion when the tips of the crutches are 6 to 8 inches to the side and in front of the foot.

Ⓟ Over time, arthritis will cause bony enlargements of the finger joints and crepitus may be felt when the patient moves the affected joint.

Ⓟ New shoes or poorly fitting shoes can cause bursitis of the heel.

Ⓟ Sexually transmitted diseases, especially gonorrhea, can contribute to joint infections with effusions.

Ⓟ Comminuted fractures result in multiple splintered bone fragments.

- ℗ A dislocation of the elbow affecting the radius and ulna usually results in significant neurovascular involvement and needs emergent reduction. A common mechanism of injury causing this dislocation is falling on outstretched hands.
- ℗ Open fractures have a higher degree of blood loss than closed fractures.
- ℗ Twisting motions cause spiral fractures. One mechanism of injury to consider is abuse.
- ℗ Front seat passengers in motor vehicle collisions may sustain hip fractures.
- ℗ Pelvic fractures carry a high mortality rate because of associated blood loss and damage to structures within and around the pelvis.
- ℗ The lower arm, hand, lower leg and foot are the most common sites of compartment syndrome.
- ℗ The earliest indicator of compartment syndrome is an aching pain in the area which is out of proportion to the injury.

Ⓟ Instruct patients to wrap cold packs before applying them to the skin to reduce cold injuries to the area.

Ⓟ The majority of low back pain is related to intervertebral disk disease.

Ⓟ Previous joint surgery or joint trauma increases the risk that the affected joint will develop an effusion.

Ⓟ Dislocations are described in terms of the distal segment in relation to the proximal segment. (E.g. – if the radius is dislocated behind the humerus, it is termed a posterior elbow dislocation.)

Ⓟ Dislocation of the radius is commonly referred to as "nursemaid's" elbow and is caused by pulling, jerking or lifting the patient (usually a child) by the lower arm.

Ⓟ Transverse fractures go straight through the bone.

Ⓟ Oblique fractures run the length of the bone.

Ⓟ Kneeling for long periods may contribute to bursitis of the knee.

ⓟ Crush injuries frequently result in compartment syndrome.

ⓟ Gouty arthritis is nine times more common in men than women.

ⓟ Immediately elevate, immobilize and apply ice to injured joints.

ⓟ A child with "nursemaid's elbow" will refuse to use the arm with limited supination, but are often able to flex and extend the elbow. Deformity may not be noticeable.

ⓟ Compression fractures usually involve the vertebrae and are the result of axial loading or reverse axial loading.

ⓟ An indication of pelvic fractures includes pain in the pelvic area, which may be elicited by putting gentle pressure on the iliac crests or gently pushing on the symphysis pubis.

ⓟ Applying external pressure over a muscle with compartment syndrome will cause the patient pain. The area will feel taut to the practitioner.

ⓟ Common causes of rhabdomyolysis include crush injuries, electrical burns and prolonged compartment syndrome.

Ⓟ Cleanse amputation stumps with normal saline, avoid bacteriostatic solutions as they can delay bone healing if they come into contact with exposed bone.

Ⓟ Clavicular fractures are associated with pneumothoraxes and hemothoraces.

Ⓟ Passive movement of an extremity that is affected with compartment syndrome will cause the patient extreme discomfort.

Ⓟ Tendinitis occurs most frequently in the shoulder, elbow, knee and heel.

Ⓟ Extreme stretching of a joint can result in synovial fluid accumulation in the joint causing a joint effusion.

Ⓟ "Nursemaid's elbow" is most common before the age of five.

Ⓟ Clavicular fractures are treated with a figure of eight support or a sling and swath dressing.

- ⓅPossible indications of pelvic fractures include paresis or hemiparesis due to nerve involvement, blood in the vagina, urinary tract or rectum or bruising of the scrotum or labia.
- ⓅParesthesias distal to a muscle compartment is one sign of compartment syndrome. This will develop after the patient experiences the pain associated with compartment syndrome.
- Ⓟ ⓅA late sign of compartment syndrome is paralysis, the patient may describe a sensation that the limb is "giving out".
- ⓅThe pain of costochondritis is usually described as sharp, pleuritic, unilateral and peristernal.
- ⓅCalcaneus fractures often occur when individuals fall from a significant height, landing on their feet. The energy is transmitted upwards and many times, the patient will also have tibial plateau fractures and compression fractures of the lumbar spine.

- Ⓟ People who fall landing on their side tend to put their hands out sustaining arm trauma. As the arm buckles, it can cause rib fractures, pulmonary trauma, and spleen or liver trauma.
- Ⓟ When people fall and land on their buttocks, the energy is transmitted to the pelvis, abdomen and chest causing severe life-threatening injuries.
- Ⓟ When teaching crutch walking, remind patients that handgrips should absorb the weight of the body; there should be no weight on the axilla.
- Ⓟ The pain of tendinitis is described as a "deep ache" worse with movement.
- Ⓟ Younger people tend to sustain shoulder dislocations, older people tend to sustain shoulder fractures.
- Ⓟ The first joint usually affected with gouty arthritis is the great toe, but as the disease progresses, it affects the insteps, ankles, heels, knees, wrists, fingers and elbows.

ⓟ The onset of pain with gouty arthritis is at night. Any clothing over the joint, movement of the joint or weight-bearing on the joint is described as intolerable pain.

ⓟ A "Y-shaped" plaster splint (sugar tong) is applied from the axilla, around the elbow and back to the shoulder for humerus fractures.

ⓟ Femur fractures are often associated with blood loss.

ⓟ Late compartment syndrome will result in a pale appearance to the affected limb. If the limb is held dependent, it will appear dusky.

ⓟ Be careful not to allow an amputated part to freeze or become frostbitten when preserving it in an ice bath.

ⓟ The last sign of compartment syndrome to develop is loss of pulse. Pressures within the affected compartment must be close to systolic pressure for this to occur.

ⓟ Radial nerve damage is a common complication of fractures of the middle or distal portion of the humerus.

Ⓟ Pressures within a muscle compartment may be measured using an intercompartmental pressure measuring device.

Ⓟ Elbow fractures frequently involve radial artery and nerve damage. Assess neurovascular status every 30 – 60 minutes.

Ⓟ Anterior dislocation of the hip results in flexion, abduction and external rotation. Posterior dislocation of the hip results in flexion, adduction, and internal rotation.

Ⓟ The pain of costochondritis is exacerbated by movement and deep inspiration.

Ⓟ Teach patients to rewrap elastic bandages twice a day and remove at night when the limb is not in a dependent position.

Ⓟ The pain of bursitis of the hip may be elicited by lying the patient on the side with the affected hip uppermost and the ipsilateral knee slightly flexed.

Ⓟ Exacerbations of gouty arthritis are usually accompanied by fever and an elevated uric acid level.

Ⓟ After joint reduction, patients need to be instructed how to minimize movement of the joint in the post-reduction period to prevent re-injuring the joint.

Ⓟ Closed reduction is usually used to treat a forearm fracture followed by application of a cast with the elbow flexed at 90 degrees.

Ⓟ Ankle fractures are associated with peroneal nerve damage.

Ⓟ Slings are applied after cast application for a forearm fracture. Patient teaching should stress the importance of not letting the hand become dependent or droop at the wrist.

Ⓟ The needle of intercompartment pressure measuring devices should not be placed through infected or contaminated tissue when measuring compartment pressures.

Ⓟ Instruct patients to elevate injured extremities above the level of the heart for the first 24 hours to reduce swelling.

Ⓟ The pain of costochondritis can be reproduced when pressure is applied to the external chest wall at the location of the inflammation.

- Ⓟ A joint effusion is painful, edematous, erythematous, hot to touch, and tender with limited range of motion.
- Ⓟ Dislocated hips should be reduced within six hours to prevent femoral head necrosis.
- Ⓟ Treatment for scaphoid fractures includes application of a spica cast.
- Ⓟ If a patient has a pelvic fracture and a traction splint increases pain after application, it should be removed.
- Ⓟ Perform a thorough neurovascular assessment prior to application of a splint. Gentle traction should be applied if neurovascular status is compromised prior to applying the splint.
- Ⓟ Perform a neurovascular assessment after splint application and if any factors have deteriorated since splint application, the splint should be removed.

- Ⓟ The needle of intercompartmental pressure measuring devices should not be inserted near the fracture site to avoid contaminating the bone ends.
- Ⓟ Patients with compartment syndrome may present with signs of dehydration and renal failure.
- Ⓟ Treatment for bursitis includes rest, ice, compression, and elevation as well as non-steroidal anti-inflammatory drugs.
- Ⓟ Patients with gouty arthritis have an increased risk of developing kidney stones.
- Ⓟ Treatment for severe bursitis includes application of a splint Bursitis of the heel may be treated with application of a moleskin to the back of the foot.
- Ⓟ Intravenous colchicine is used to reduce the inflammation of gout along with non-steroidal anti-inflammatory drugs.
- Ⓟ Patellar dislocations are immobilized with a cast or splint after reduction.

Ⓟ Cover an open wound with a sterile dressing prior to applying a splint to the area.

Ⓟ Remove all external sources of external pressure (splints, elastic bandages, heavy blankets) from a limb that is suspected of being affected by compartment syndrome.

Ⓟ Abnormal laboratory studies associated with rhabdomyolysis include hypocalcemia, hyperkalemia, hyperuricemia, and increased creatinine phosphokinase.

Ⓟ Severe cases of bursitis may require bursal aspiration or even an incision and drainage in the presence of infection.

Ⓟ A radial or ulnar gutter splint is applied with the metacarpal joints flexed 70 to 90 degrees and the wrist extended 20 degrees for metacarpal fractures.

Ⓟ Femur fractures may involve injury to the peroneal nerve, sciatic nerve and popliteal artery.

- Ⓟ Common manifestations of hip fractures include severe pain with movement of the leg, shortening of the extremity and external rotation.
- Ⓟ Do not elevate or allow a limb to be in the dependent position when compartment syndrome is suspected. Instead, the limb should be kept at the level of the heart.
- Ⓟ Treat patients with pelvic fractures as major trauma patients. Apply high flow oxygen, initiate of two large bore intravenous lines and draw blood for type and cross.
- Ⓟ Fasciotomies may be required for severe compartment syndrome.
- Ⓟ Patients with fractures of the greater trochanter may be able to ambulate, although they will usually experience pain when they do so.
- Ⓟ A white blood cell count above 100,000 in the specimen removed during arthrocentesis for a joint effusion indicates an infectious process in the joint.

Ⓟ A white blood cell count less than 60,000 in the specimen removed during arthrocentesis for a joint effusion is more indicative of an inflammatory process.

Ⓟ Patients with pelvic fractures frequently find flexion of the knees is more comfortable. Flexion of the knees increases intracranial pressure and should be withheld if the patient also has a head injury.

Ⓟ When teaching patients to go up stairs with crutches, the uninjured leg goes up the step first, followed by the injured leg and crutches.

Ⓟ Costochondritis is treated with non-steroidal anti-inflammatory drugs.

Ⓟ Nerve involvement with low back pain can cause foot drop, altered gait, altered deep tendon reflexes, loss of sharp-dull discrimination, altered bowel, bladder and sexual function.

Ⓟ Steroids may be injected into severely inflamed joints affected by gout to reduce inflammation.

Ⓟ Discharge teaching for patients with costochondritis includes the importance of deep breathing to prevent respiratory complications and avoidance of exertional activities.

Ⓟ Substances which can induce an attack of gouty arthritis include thiazide diuretics, alcohol, and foods high in purine (herring, mussels, yeast, salmon, sardines, anchovies, veal, bacon and organ meats).

Ⓟ An area of tendinitis appears swollen, and tenderness is noted when pressure is applied in a rolling motion over the affected tendon.

Ⓟ Dislocation of the knee is rare but is usually associated with peroneal nerve and popliteal artery damage.

Ⓟ Non-displaced tibia and fibula fractures are placed in a long leg splint or cast. Unstable or displaced fractures usually require surgery.

- ℗ When possible, clothing and footwear should be removed before application of a traction splint.
- ℗ Volkmann's contracture is a permanent disability resulting from prolonged ischemia secondary to compartment syndrome or impingement of the radial nerve.
- ℗ Depending on the severity of the fracture, broken ankles will require either application of a walking cast or open reduction and fixation.
- ℗ Wrap amputated parts in sterile gauze moistened with normal saline or lactated Ringer's solution, then place in a sealed plastic bag and place the bag in ice water.
- ℗ Patients with rhabdomyolysis will have dark brown urine, general malaise, fever and muscle tenderness.
- ℗ Indications of Volkmann's contracture include inability to move the digits distal to the injury and severe pain when those digits are manipulated.

- Ⓟ All bony prominences and wounds should be padded prior to splint application.
- Ⓟ Steroidal injections into the bursal sac are sometimes used to reduce edema in overuse bursitis.
- Ⓟ Patients with dislocated knees will be unable to straighten their leg.
- Ⓟ Probenecid and Sulfinpyrazone (Anturane) may promote excretion of uric acid to decrease the effects of gouty arthritis.
- Ⓟ Tibial fractures frequently occur with knee dislocations.
- Ⓟ A Volkmann's contracture is a possible complication of a supracondylar fracture.
- Ⓟ Knee dislocations usually require admission.
- Ⓟ Aspirin interferes with excretion of uric acid and should be avoided in patients with gout.
- Ⓟ When teaching patients to go down stairs with crutches, the crutches go down the steps first, and then both the injured and uninjured leg follows through.

- ℗ Patients with ankle dislocations frequently have associated fractures. A splint will be applied followed by open reduction.
- ℗ When possible, splints should immobilize joints above and below the level of the injury.
- ℗ Patients with back pain should be encouraged to put a small towel roll under the lower back when lying flat to increase comfort.
- ℗ Patients with rhabdomyolysis require large volumes of intravenous fluids to maintain kidney function. Sodium bicarbonate will also help prevent renal failure in these cases.
- ℗ Pelvic splints or binders should be promptly applied to pelvic fractures to increase comfort and decrease bleeding.
- ℗ Always assess neurovascular status before and after applying a traction splint.
- ℗ Immediate return of blood to a nail bed after blanching is considered a normal finding when testing capillary refill. If it takes two seconds or longer for refill, it is considered an abnormal finding.

- ℗ Allopurinal may decrease the production of uric acid and reduce attacks of gouty arthritis.
- ℗ Tendinitis is treated with non-steroidal anti-inflammatory medications; compressive dressings, elevation and physical therapy for severe cases.
- ℗ Joints which have been reduced will usually be placed in immobilization devices and slings applied when appropriate.
- ℗ When applying a traction splint over an open fracture, do not place straps over an open wound.
- ℗ The fluid of a joint effusion may be removed with arthrocentesis.
- ℗ If a pulse cannot be easily palpated, consider using a Doppler.
- ℗ Splints are applied with the limb in a position of function.
- ℗ Do not wrap amputated parts in water for preservation, as water is hypo-osmolar and can damage tissues.

Ⓟ When applying tourniquets, consider the "rule of twos". Apply the tourniquet two inches above the stump or bleeding area, make sure the tourniquet is a minimum of two inches wide and apply a second tourniquet two inches above the first if the first tourniquet does not adequately control bleeding.

Ⓟ Place an amputated part in a cooler that is filled half with ice and half with water for best preservation.

Ⓟ Amputated tissue is best preserved at 4 degrees Celsius.

Ⓟ Common complications of clavicular and scapular fractures include injuries to the large vessels, pulmonary injuries, rib fractures and cervical spinal fractures.

Ⓟ It takes significant force to fracture the scapula. Scapular fractures may also cause injuries to the brachial plexus, the spleen and the humerus.

Ⓟ The treatment for clavicular and scapular fractures is the application of a sling and resting the affected side.

- Ⓟ A Monteggia's fracture is associated with falling on an outstretched hand. It causes a fracture of the distal one-third of the ulna with an associated radial head dislocation.
- Ⓟ A nightstick fracture occurs when an individual tries to block a blow with the forearm causing a fracture of the midshaft of the ulna (but the radius is unbroken)
- Ⓟ An appropriately placed pelvic sling is applied across the greater trochanters and the symphysis pubis. It should cause internal rotation of the lower limbs.
- Ⓟ A pelvic binder will tamponade venous bleeding in the pelvis but does little to stop arterial bleeding. If, after application of the pelvic binder, the patient's hemodynamic status does not improve, surgery will likely be required.
- Ⓟ Aggressive fluid resuscitation is often needed for patients with pelvic fractures.

- ℗ Causes of an Achilles tendon rupture include forced plantar flexion of the foot or unexpected dorsiflexion of the foot.
- ℗ Fluoroquinolone medications (e.g. Levaquin, Cipro, Avelox) weaken tendons and may be associated with tendon injuries.
- ℗ When the Achilles tendon ruptures, the patient may feel a sharp pain or "pop" in the heal. The arch of the foot will flatten and the patient will be unable to stand on the ball of the foot or plantar flex the foot.
- ℗ ED treatment of an Achille's tendon rupture is usually to splint the foot in plantar flexion, provide crutches and ensure the patient follows up with an orthopedic specialist.
- ℗ Patients with calcaneus fractures will often complain of pain when the foot is hyperflexed.
- ℗ ED treatment for a calcaneus fracture is the application of a compression dressing, crutches and encouragement to follow up with an orthopedic specialist for definitive repair.

Ⓟ Avoid movement of an injured extremity and apply splints to fractures to reduce the incidence of bleeding in the area and the occurrence of a fat emboli.

Ⓟ Elevate injured extremities above the level of the heart to reduce edema unless compartment syndrome is suspected. In that case, the limb should be kept AT the level of the heart.

Ⓟ Protect the skin from frost bite when applying ice over an orthopedic injury.

Ⓟ Cover open fractures with saline soaked dressings.

References for orthopedic emergencies

Drew, B., Bennett, B. L., & Littlejohn, L. (2014). Application of Current Hemorrhage Control Techniques for Backcountry Care: Part One, Tourniquets and Hemorrhage Control Adjuncts. *Wilderness and Environmental Medicine*, 1 - 10.

Halpern J.S. (2013). Musculoskeletal Trauma. In B. B. Hammond, & P. Gerber-Zimmerman (Eds.), *Sheehy's Emergency Nursing: Principals and Practice* (7 ed., pp. 427 - 437). Philadelphia: Elsevier.

Harris, C (2013). Abdominal Trauma. In B. B. Hammond, & P. Gerber-Zimmerman (Eds.), *Sheehy's Emergency Nursing: Principals and Practice* (7 ed., pp. 419 - 425). Philadelphia: Elsevier.

Ledgerwood, A. M., & Lucas, C. E. (2014). The Management of Extremity Compartment Syndrome. In J. L. Cameron, & A. M. Cameron, *Current Surgical Therapy* (11 ed., pp. 1124 - 1128). Philadelphia: Elsevier.

Melendez, T. (2013). *Musculoskeletal Injuries*. Retrieved January 2016, 2016, from University of California - Los Angeles: https://www.cpc.mednet.ucla.edu/sites/default/files/Refresher131112/Day1/Transition/Musculo-skeletalInjuries.pdf

Moore, D. (n.d.). Management of Amputations. In J. R. Roberts, *Roberts and Hedges Clinical Procedures in Emergency Medicine* (6 ed., pp. 923 - 930). Philadelphia: Elsevier.

Pallin, D. J. (2014). Knee and Lower Leg. In J. A. Marx, R. S. Hockberger, & R. M. Walls, *Rosen's Emergency Medicine* (8 ed., pp. 698-722). Philadelphia: Elsevier.

Patterson, L. A. (2013). Pelvic Fractures. In J. G. Adams, *Emergency Medicine* (2 ed., pp. 710 - 715). Philadelphia: Elsevier.

Schrank, K. S. (2013). Joint Disorders. In J. G. Adams, *Emergency Medicine* (2 ed., pp. 929 - 943). Philadelphia: Elsevier.

Solheim J. (2013). Assessment and Stabilization of the Trauma Patient. In B. B. Hammond, & P. Gerber-Zimmerman (Eds.), *Sheehy's Emergency Nursing: Principals and Practice* (7 ed., pp. 369 - 377). Philadelphia: Elsevier.

Williams, D. T., & Kim, H. T. (2014). Wrist and Forearm. In J. A. Marx, R. S. Hockberger, & R. M. Walls, *Rosen's Emergency Medicine* (8 ed., pp. 570 - 595). Philadelphia: Elsevier.

Wood, G. W. (2013). General Principles of Fracture Treatment. In S. T. Canale, & J. H. Beaty, *Campbell's Operative Orthopaedics* (12 ed., pp. 2560 - 2615). Philadelphia: Elsevier.

Wound
Emergencies

- ℗ Wounds caused by compressive forces are more susceptible to infection.
- ℗ Blunt trauma occurs when energy is transferred to the body without penetrating the skin.
- ℗ Penetrating trauma occurs when the injuring instrument penetrates the skin.
- ℗ Closure by primary intention is bringing the wound edges together with sutures, staples, steri-strips, wound glue or other materials shortly after the injury.
- ℗ Human bites carry a very high risk of infection, including infection with Hepatitis B.
- ℗ A contusion is a collection of blood under the skin.
- ℗ A hematoma is a significant collection of blood that clots.
- ℗ Dark, oozing blood is indicative of venous bleeding, bright red, pulsating blood is indicative of arterial bleeding.

- Ⓟ Closure by secondary intention is allowing the wound to close by granulation without intervention.
- Ⓟ Human wounds should receive copious irrigation and debridement of devitalized tissue to prevent infection.
- Ⓟ Lidocaine <u>with</u> epinephrine is usually chosen as a local anesthetic to close highly vascular areas to decrease bleeding around the wound.
- Ⓟ Lidocaine <u>without</u> epinephrine should be used to close wounds on the nose, penis, ears or digits.
- Ⓟ Patients should be taught to apply sun block with sun protection factor (SPF) of at least 15 to wounds for at least six months to prevent discoloration of the area as it heals.
- Ⓟ Remove body jewelry from infected wound piercing sites.
- Ⓟ Patients should be instructed to leave tape closures in place until they fall off.

- Ⓟ Patients on immunosuppressive drugs have increased risk of infection after injury.
- Ⓟ Factors which can delay wound healing include diabetes, long-term steroid use, poor tissue perfusion in the area of the wound, obesity, malnutrition, aging and anemia.
- Ⓟ Closure by secondary intention is reserved for wounds with devitalized tissue, severely contaminated wounds or wounds that are obviously infected.
- Ⓟ Mixing sodium bicarbonate 8.4% (Neut) with lidocaine or warming lidocaine by running the vial under warm water decreases the pain associated with infiltration.
- Ⓟ Human bite wounds are usually left open to close by secondary intention. A bulky dressing is applied to minimize movement.
- Ⓟ Patients with host immunocompromise such as HIV/AIDS and neutropenia are at risk of delayed wound healing.

- ℗ The longer the time between occurrence of a wound and treatment for the wound, the more likely there will be delays in wound healing.
- ℗ Petroleum jelly or acetone can be used to remove wound glue which has stuck in ways that it was not intended.
- ℗ Dressings should be maintained over a wound for at least 48 hours after closure.
- ℗ For sutures in the eyelids, lips and face; patients should be taught to return in 3 to 5 days for removal.
- ℗ For sutures in the eyebrows, patients should be taught to return in 4 to 5 days for removal.
- ℗ For sutures in the ear, patients should be taught to return in 4 to 6 days for removal.
- ℗ For sutures in the scalp, trunk, hands and feet, patients should be taught to return in 7 to 10 days for removal.

- Ⓟ For sutures in the arms and legs, patients should be taught to return in 10 to 14 days for removal.
- Ⓟ For sutures over joints, patients should be taught to return in 14 days for removal.
- Ⓟ Patients should be instructed to have staples removed in 10 to 14 days.
- Ⓟ Hollow point bullets tend to create greater injury then full metal jacket bullets.
- Ⓟ A stage one pressure ulcer is one in which the skin is reddened, but the skin is unbroken. The redness will usually fade when pressure is relieved on the area.
- Ⓟ Treatment for a stage one pressure ulcer includes turning the patient, alleviating pressure to the area; covering, protecting or cushioning the area.
- Ⓟ Primary injuries in an explosion are created from an expanding wall of gas that extends from the blast.

Ⓟ Primary injuries from an explosion usually affect gas filled organs and include ruptured tympanic membranes, air emboli and gastric or intestinal ruptures.

Ⓟ Cat bites carry a very high risk of infection because of the deep puncture wounds caused by their long fangs.

Ⓟ Long-term steroid use may cause a delay in wound healing.

Ⓟ Saline and betadine are frequently chosen for wound care and irrigation.

Ⓟ Tape closure carries a lower risk of infection than sutures.

Ⓟ Hydrogen peroxide is not recommended for wound care because it causes absorption of oxygen into the wound, increases cell destruction, and does not protect against anaerobes.

Ⓟ Tape closure is reserved for superficial linear wounds under minimal tension.

Ⓟ An abrasion is defined as removal of the epithelium with exposure of either the dermis or subcutaneous layer.

Ⓟ Common combinations of topical anesthetics include Tetracaine, adrenalin and cocaine (TAC), Xylocaine, adrenalin and pontacaine (XAP) and Lidocaine, epinephrine and tetracaine (LET).

Ⓟ Patients sent home with a puncture wound should be instructed to soak the wound in warm soapy water two or three times per day for two to four days.

Ⓟ Prophylactic antibiotics should be given to patients with human bite wounds within three hours of arrival to the ED.

Ⓟ Wounds that are grossly contaminated should be irrigated for at least five minutes.

Ⓟ Tape closure is not recommended for wounds that are likely to become edematous.

Ⓟ To apply a topical anesthetic, saturate a cotton ball with the solution, place it over the wound and cover with a tegaderm dressing. It should be left in place a minimum of 20 minutes.

Ⓟ Surgicel or Gelfoam may be used on an avulsion to control bleeding.

- ⓟ Wounds caused by high pressure products (e.g. paint or grease guns) usually require surgical debridement and extensive irrigation, often under general anesthetic.
- ⓟ Wounds to the knuckles of the dorsum of the hand caused by punching someone in the mouth carry a high risk of joint effusions and osteomyelitis.
- ⓟ Abrasions covering a large surface area may result in significant fluid loss that will require fluid resuscitation.
- ⓟ Debris imbedded in abrasions must be removed within four to six hours on the extremities and eight hours on the face to prevent permanent tattooing in the area.
- ⓟ Soaps with strong cleaning agents or those containing alcohols are avoided when performing wound care as they may cause further tissue damage.
- ⓟ Secondary injuries from an explosion are created by pieces of debris that fly from the blast site and include lacerations and impaled objects.

- Ⓟ Excessive hair around a wound should be clipped, but not shaved, to reduce the risk of infection.
- Ⓟ Dog bites are associated with underlying crush injuries.
- Ⓟ Tincture of benzoin applied to wound edges before application of tape increases adherence of the tape.
- Ⓟ Wound glue forms a thin waterproof bandage in one second on moist skin and several seconds on dry skin.
- Ⓟ Wounds caused by high pressure products (e.g. grease or paint guns) inject substances that separate fascial planes, neurovascular bundles and tendon sheaths.   These need emergent treatment.
- Ⓟ Vegetative matter (e.g. wood or thorns) in a wound may require computerized tomography, sonography, fluoroscopy, or local would exploration to find and remove.
- Ⓟ An avulsion is defined as full-thickness tissue loss that prevents wound edge approximation.

- Ⓟ A degloving is a form of avulsion in which the full thickness of skin is peeled away from the underling tissue.
- Ⓟ Antibiotic ointment should not be applied to wounds that will be closed using tape as this will decrease tape adherence.
- Ⓟ A stage two pressure ulcer is one in which the skin has broken over the area. It may appear as a broken or unbroken blister.
- Ⓟ Treatment for a stage two pressure ulcer includes cleaning and covering the area with dressings designed to insulate and absorb as well as protect the area.
- Ⓟ Topical cocaine solutions may cause central nervous system stimulation and vasomotor collapse.
- Ⓟ *Pasteurella multicodia* is commonly found in the saliva of cats and can cause cellulitis, osteomyelitis, pleuritis, septic arthritis and bacteremia in the affected area.
- Ⓟ The cosmetic result with staple closure is less desirable than with suturing.

- Ⓟ Tertiary injuries in an explosion are caused by bodies being hurled through the air by the explosion and include blunt injuries as the body strikes various objects.
- Ⓟ Patients being discharged home after wound closure should be instructed to elevate the affected part for 48 hours to minimize pain and swelling.
- Ⓟ Patients with foreign bodies imbedded in their wounds have higher rates of infection.
- Ⓟ Blood loss due to difficult hemostasis is a common problem associated with avulsion injuries.
- Ⓟ Eyebrows should never be shaved as they may not grow back. They also serve as a landmark for wound alignment during closure.
- Ⓟ Small avulsion injuries may heal by secondary intention, large avulsions often require skin grafts.
- Ⓟ A puncture wound is one whose depth is greater than the surface of the wound.

- ⓟ Staples do not provide as much hemostasis as sutures but have decreased infection rates.
- ⓟ To perform a local nerve block, or digital block, an anesthetic agent is injected directly along the nerve where anesthesia is required.
- ⓟ Abrasions are covered with ointment after cleansing to prevent infection after which a non-adhering dressing should be applied.
- ⓟ If vegetative matter (e.g. wood or thorns) is suspected in a wound, do NOT soak the area to prevent the vegetative matter from absorbing the fluid and disintegrating.
- ⓟ Puncture wounds tend to seal off quickly and bleed less, preventing bacteria from exiting the wound, therefore, they carry a high risk of infection.
- ⓟ A stage three pressure ulcer is one which extends through all layers of the skin resulting in a wound with high risk for infection.

℗ Treatment for a stage three pressure ulcer includes alleviating pressure from the area, protecting it from infection and considering a referral to a wound care specialist.

℗ Viscous lidocaine may be applied to abrasions before vigorous cleaning.

℗ Staples are used to close linear wounds on the scalp, trunk and extremities.

℗ Anesthetic is rarely used when stapling a wound if two or less staples are anticipated.

℗ Wound glue has a lower infection rate than sutures.

℗ Topical lidocaine will cause a white ring around the area of application due to vasoconstriction.

℗ Petroleum (Vaseline), Xeroform gauze or other nonadhering material and pressure dressings (as needed) are placed over avulsions.

Ⓟ To perform a Bier block, a tourniquet is applied above the repair site, the anesthetic agent is injected distal to the wound, and the tourniquet is left in place until the repair is done.

Ⓟ Puncture wounds near joint spaces have a high rate of bacterial inoculation into the joint space that can lead to joint sepsis.

Ⓟ Wound glue should not be used on wounds in areas of high tension such as near joints.

Ⓟ Patients with increasing pain in the foot after a puncture wound to the bottom of the foot should be instructed to seek medical treatment because of the high risk of osteomyelitis with these injuries.

Ⓟ Puncture wounds on the bottom of the foot have a high rate of tarsal bone osteomyelitis because body weight forces the object into the bones.

Ⓟ Because of the high risk of infection, puncture wounds should be soaked for 10 – 15 minutes.

Ⓟ Non-puncture wounds should be cleansed rather than soaked.

Ⓟ Bites at risk for infection (those involving joints, ligaments, tendons and bones as well as those to the hand and foot) may be left to close by secondary intention to decrease infection.

Ⓟ Patients who have wound glue applied should be taught to avoid applying liquids or ointment to the closed wound because it can weaken the glue.

Ⓟ Animal bites more than 12 hours old are likely to be left open to close by secondary intention to decrease the risk of infection.

Ⓟ A stage four pressure ulcer is one which extends not only through every layer of the skin, but into underlying muscle, tendons and bone resulting in the potential for life-threatening infections.

Ⓟ Treatment for a stage four pressure ulcer may include surgical removal of necrotic or decayed tissue. A wound care referral is always warranted.

Ⓟ The faster a bullet is moving as it strikes a patient, the greater the risk of injury.

- Ⓟ As a bullet passes through tissue, it takes tissue along with it causing what is called the "permanent cavity".
- Ⓟ Faster moving bullets will displace tissue laterally away from the permanent cavity creating a temporary cavity. Although the tissue displaced by the moving bullet returns to its original position, it leaves blunt trauma known as the "temporary cavity".
- Ⓟ Very fast moving bullets create pressure waves that progress outwards away from the permanent cavity causing injury to hollow organs far away from the actual trajectory of the bullet.
- Ⓟ Large abrasions carry a high risk for evaporative heat and fluid loss. Keep the patient warm and provide fluids to combat these complications.
- Ⓟ The longer the barrel of a firearm from which a bullet is fired, the faster the bullet will move and the greater the injury potential.
- Ⓟ The caliber of a bullet is the diameter of the bullet at its leading edge. It is measured in 1/100ths of an inch.

ⓟ Glass and metal in wounds can be visualized with an x-ray.

ⓟ Hair removal around wounds should be avoided when possible. If hair removal is necessary, it should be accomplished with scissors or clippers rather than shaving.

ⓟ Wounds that carry a high risk for tetanus include those obviously contaminated with dirt, feces, soil, saliva as well as puncture wounds, avulsions, wounds resulting from missiles, crushing, burns and frostbite.

ⓟ If a patient has not been fully immunized for tetanus prior to an ED visit and the patient has a wound that carries a high risk for tetanus, the patient should receive both Tdap and tetanus immune globulin during the ED visit.

ⓟ If patients are not fully immunized for tetanus prior to an ED visit and receive a dose of Tdap, the patient should be encouraged to obtain to further tetanus immunizations for full immunity.

- ⓟ Tetanus is a serious disease that causes painful tightening of the muscles. The bacteria is found in soil as well as the intestine of animals and humans.
- ⓟ Tetanus infections peak in the summer or wet season.
- ⓟ A contusion is caused by the rupture of blood vessels with extravasation of erythrocytes.
- ⓟ A hematoma is caused by the rupture of an artery or vein and will continue to expand until the pressure in the tissue exceeds the pressure in an artery or vein.
- ⓟ Because blood sets up a foci for infection, wounds near a hematoma or contusion carries higher risks for infections.

Bibliography for wound emergencies

Williams, D. T., & Kim, H. T. (2014). Wrist and Forearm. In J. A. Marx, R. S. Hockberger, & R. M. Walls, *Rosen's Emergency Medicine* (8 ed., pp. 570 - 595). Philadelphia: Elsevier.

Pallin, D. J. (2014). Knee and Lower Leg. In J. A. Marx, R. S. Hockberger, & R. M. Walls, *Rosen's Emergency Medicine* (8 ed., pp. 698-722). Philadelphia: Elsevier.

Herr, R D. (2013). Wound Management. In B. B. Hammond, & P. Gerber-Zimmerman (Eds.), *Sheehy's Emergency Nursing: Principals and Practice* (7 ed., pp. 147 - 160). Philadelphia: Elsevier.

Mootrey, G., Tiwari, T., & Weinbaum, C. (2015). Tetanus. *Epidemiology and Prevention of Vaccine-Preventable Diseases*, pp. 341 - 352. Retrieved from http://www.cdc.gov/vaccines/pubs/pinkbook/index.html

National Pressure Ulcer Advisory Panel. (No Date). *NPUAP Pressure Ulcer Stages/Category*. Retrieved from National Pressure Ulcer Advisory Panel: http://www.npuap.org/resources/educational-and-clinical-resources/npuap-pressure-ulcer-stagescategories/